Heal.thy Low-Back

Release Low-Back Pain by
Understanding the Cause and the Cure

Michelle Andrie

ISBN-13: 978-1-958848-53-1 print edition
ISBN-13: 978-1-958848-54-8 e-book edition

Waterside Productions

2055 Oxford Ave
Cardiff, CA 92007
www.waterside.com

To all of my teachers

Table of Contents

Introduction vii

Part I: The Cause of Low-Back Pain - Awareness. 1
Chapter 1 - A Whole Body Challenge. 3
Chapter 2 - The Four Roots of Low-Back Pain 9
Chapter 3 - Low-Back Pain Self-Assessment. 17

Part II: The Cause of Low-Back Pain - Digging Deeper 27
Chapter 4 - What Is Fascia? 29
Chapter 5 - Fascia + Muscle Move Bone 35
Chapter 6 - You Are an Energy Body 39
Chapter 7 - Posture of Pain 47

Part III: The Cure – Your Daily Practice 51
Chapter 8 - The Way Out of Low-Back Pain. 53
Chapter 9 - The Pain-Free Low-Back Posture 59

Part III: The Cure – Create Your NEW Pain-Free
        Low-Back Posture 65
Chapter 10 - Release Your Feet, Legs, and Anger to
        Form a Strong Foundation 67
Chapter 11 - Let Go of Your Hips, Glutes, Piriformis, and
        Control to Create Stability 87
Chapter 12 - Free Fear From Your Quads and Iliopsoas to
        Connect to Your Emotional Guidance System 101

Chapter 13 - Power Your Core and Strenthen Your Belly 135
Chapter 14 - Releasing Sciatica 165
Chapter 15 - Releasing Sacroiliac Joint Problems 171

Part IV: The Cure For Low-Back Pain – Maintenance 177
Chapter 16 - How to Get Out of Low-Back Pain -
        Your Daily Practice 179
Chapter 17 - How to Stay Out of Low-Back Pain
        Facing Life Challenges 197

References: 203

Introduction

If you are alive, you can heal.

For many of us, the journey out of low-back pain is a long, painful, difficult, and expensive one. It can be incredibly frustrating because most people seeking a solution to their low-back pain spend much time and money in the traditional medical world without receiving substantial relief.

I too spent years seeking help from the doctors and physical therapists with whom I worked at Presbyterian Hospital in Dallas, Texas. I took their advice and tried the pills, injections, and exercises; only stopping when they suggested surgery because I knew that surgery had only a 50% success rate – and of the 50% that found relief with surgery, it was only temporary. Their low-back pain came back over time.

While I was attempting to find a cure in the traditional medical community, I searched out every yoga remedy, got popped and twisted by chiropractors, poked with needles by acupuncturists, had my mind probed in psychotherapy, took many supplements, became a raw foodie and bared my soul to spiritual teachers.

And still, my low-back pain persisted.
I was a Yoga Therapist working in a hospital helping others face their challenges and I couldn't help myself.

I felt hopeless.
All I wanted to do was get back to swimming, hiking, practicing yoga, playing with my daughter, enjoying my friends, cooking

dinner, redoing my old farmhouse, gardening, and working with my yoga therapy clients – without low-back pain.

Can you relate?
Do you want to get out of low-back pain and get back to doing all of the things you love to do?

Well, I have good news for you!!
As I write this, I am completely free from low-back pain and have been for nearly two decades. If I can get out of low-back pain after fifteen years of suffering, you can too!

My Low-Back Pain Story
I remember hitting the lowest point in my long journey with chronic low-back pain. I woke up in the middle of the night feeling the familiar stabbing back pain and lay there attempting to catch my breath. I knew if I moved, the pain would only get worse because this had happened to me so many times before.

I started crying, then sobbing uncontrollably. I didn't want to live with this kind of pain anymore. My partner heard my cries and got out of bed to help me to my yoga mat which lived at the end of our bed because these late-night low-back pain episodes happened regularly.

I lay on my mat, tears running down my face, thinking … My BACK is in too much pain. It had seized up for the millionth time a few days prior for no good reason at all. I could barely move and care for myself; let alone the house, my partner, or my kid. And now this stabbing pain was keeping me from even resting?

I couldn't even get out of bed by myself. That was the worst feeling. I felt like a burden, a complete FAILURE.

Why me??

I had been suffering from low-back pain for about thirteen years at that point. I thought that I was doing everything right – I was a yoga therapist for goodness sake!! As I shared, I had already seen every specialist and was doing everything I could think of to just get some relief. Yet my low-back pain persisted. Not one of the countless doctors or healers whom I'd seen was able to give me lasting solutions.

My life was passing me by. I was living with chronic pain every single day which became so debilitating several times a year that I couldn't even get out of bed by myself. I couldn't take living like this anymore.

At that moment on the floor, I decided to give up any hope of finding a solution and accept my fate. I truly believed that I was destined to live with low-back pain for the rest of my life.

But then a very small miracle occurred. My hand brushed the golf ball my dog had been playing with earlier that evening. I grabbed it and placed it under my right butt cheek. And just like that, I felt a bit of relief. I lay there rolling on my butt cheek for several minutes – long enough that I could begin to move on my own. Amazingly, I was then able to get up and put myself back to bed.

I lay there puzzling over this miracle. What had happened?

Even a hint of some kind of improvement galvanized me. I had to know more! So I took myself on a journey to learn about it. That moment of relief led me to study a little-known part of the body that connects the body and the mind and contracts or releases muscles, the fascia.

Ultimately, these studies led me to many teachers; all of whom helped me to better understand my body, my energy flow, my emotions, and my mindset. My long journey culminated in an amazing discovery: this one magical system, the fascia, that I knew nothing about, but quickly realized was the key to healing my low-back pain.

During this journey, I put together a natural healing method that gave me lasting low-back pain relief. I still remember waking up one morning after a good night's sleep and realizing that I hadn't felt pain in my lower back in days.

It truly was a miracle!

Remember … my life experience included feeling low-back pain EVERY SINGLE DAY … for years. Slowly I found that I was able to move, bend over, pick up things, walk, sit, and cook dinner – ALL WITHOUT low-back PAIN!!

I had finally found the solution I'd been searching for! And it wasn't even that hard! Better yet, it didn't involve drugs, surgery, endless visits to the chiropractor, massage, or relying on anyone else to "fix" me. The discoveries I made from that initial late-night "A-ha moment" were so exciting that I began to practice them on my low-back clients.

Hi, My name is Michelle Andrie, a Yoga Therapist of thirty-three years, a Myofascial Release Therapist, and an expert in the energy body. In the nineteen years since my discovery, I've helped thousands of clients release low-back pain.

And now I've been led to write this book. I wanted to put my practices into one simple, accessible guide. So many people whom I've treated are now finally enjoying life again... and I want to spread this knowledge to as many people as possible.

I was able to heal my back NATURALLY without doctor visits and once again resume a happy life full of activities like swimming in the ocean. Most importantly, I now savor the gift of feeling safe, strong, and capable in my own body. This is what I hope to do for my readers.

But I need to tell you... This book is NOT for EVERYONE.

This book is for:

- People whose back pain limits their ability to do the things they love.
- Those who have lived with chronic, persistent low-back pain.
- Those who have already tried doctors, chiropractors, physical therapy, massage, acupuncture, pills, surgery, or injections... and still haven't gotten the results they want.
- Those who are ready to take 100% responsibility for their results by investing the time to create a healthy low-back.

A life of FREEDOM FROM CHRONIC BACK PAIN is possible! No need to wait and hope things get better. The time to take ACTION is NOW!

This book is a workbook. Write your answers to the questions in it, underline anything that resonates and earmark pages that you want to go back to.

Let's get you out of low-back pain!

Michelle Andrie

Part I: The Cause of Low-Back Pain - Awareness

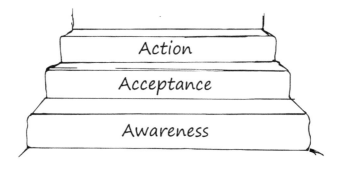

There are three steps to healing – the first one is Awareness.

Chapter 1 - A Whole Body Challenge

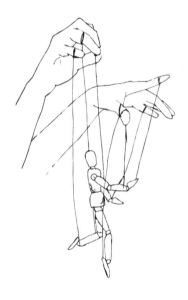

Choose or be a life
Puppet on a string is you
Unless you say no
Haiku 21/4/2b by MCW

You are merely a puppet on a string. Yes, a puppet master is at work pulling on these strings to create the posture you currently live in. This posture is what is causing your low-back pain. It is that simple.

Who, you may be asking, is the puppet master?

The puppet master pulling your strings and creating your low-back pain posture is a combination of your mind, your emotions, your memories, and your physical reactions.

In other words, you are a whole body and everything that you think, feel, remember, react to, or happens to you or around you impacts you. The body then activates specific strings in an attempt to protect you. Unfortunately, instead of protecting you, these "held pulls" ultimately only hurt you.

OK, then.... *What* are your puppet strings?

They are fascia. Everything in your body is encased in fascia, which is connective tissue. Fascinatingly enough, research has proven that fascia contains brain cells; it is fascia that responds and reacts to everything that you are experiencing.

It is fascia that creates a pull in one muscle and a release in another to form any posture where your low-back is no longer supported, compressed, shifted out of alignment, or all of these things at the same time.

We'll be diving deep into your whole body and how it works, as well as the fascia, to help you gain an understanding of your puppet master (thoughts, memories, emotions, and reactions) and the strings (fascia) that are constantly being pulled.

For now, let's discuss the whole body puppet master, the fascia strings, and how they affect the low-back.

An Experience:

Let's say that one part of your body grows tight, gets knotted up or is held in a certain position based on a thought, feeling, or reaction. Your low-back is impacted because it is located right in the center of your body. In other words, it is directly impacted by all body pulls – from your lower body (the hips, legs, and feet) and the upper body (your belly, heart, neck, and head).

For example, when your right shoulder grows tight, it will draw the whole right side of your body up and compress the lower back on the left side.

Try it.

Stand up and lift your right shoulder up and in toward your right ear. As you hold this position, notice the lift of the right side of your body and the contraction and compression that happens in your left low-back.

Did you feel that?

We all experience daily chronic lifts and holds in our bodies, all of which have an impact on the rest of the body. Most importantly, for those of us reading this book, they affect the lower back.

Let's try a hold in the lower body.

Stand up with your feet about a foot apart, and roll your left inner leg out so you are duck-footed on your left side. Make sure your right foot is facing straight ahead, not ducking out or turning in. This will cause the left hip to dip down more than the right and compress the left side of your low-back.

Try it.

Pretty wild, right?

I'm sure you noticed that the right upper shoulder pull and the turnout of the left leg both impacted your low-back.

Again, this is because your low-back is caught in the middle of the upper and lower bodies and takes the impact of all twists, pulls, or imbalances that occur above or below.

No wonder the statistics show that low-back pain is one of the most common medical ailments, with 80% of adults in the western world experiencing it at some point during their lifetime.

Now, going deeper into your whole body meaning: Let's consider you as a physical, mental, emotional, energetic, and spiritual being and examine how each of those aspects of yourself connects and impacts one another. Your right shoulder wouldn't just lift and hold on its own for no reason; it lifts for physical challenges, mental issues, emotional imbalances, energetic blocks, troubling memories, or spiritual struggles.

Let's take the example of your right shoulder lifting. It could lift because you are:

- Habitually carrying a heavy bag on your right shoulder.
- Taking on responsibility for others.
- Caretaking others too much.
- Protecting your heart from being rejected or hurt by others.
- Grieving the loss of someone.
- Living with troubling memories around loving someone.
- Struggling with your faith or trust.

You could lift your right shoulder for one of the reasons above, a combination of several, or all of the above. In other words, we are a complex system that is affected by our physical, mental, emotional, and spiritual challenges.

Now let's take the second example, of the left inner leg turning out. It could turn out because you are:

- Gripping your left butt cheek.
- Controlling others.
- Wishing something inside of yourself was different than it is.
- Impacted by the genetics and DNA from your mother's side of the family.
- Operating out of the childhood teachings from your mom.
- Unwilling to let emotions flow.

Again, you could turn your left leg and foot out for one of the reasons above, a combination of several, or all the above. Again, we are a complex system that is affected by all of our thoughts, beliefs, memories, and reactions. To make matters even more challenging, we hold on to things that happened in the past and are often posturing ourselves based on those memories.

To top that off, researchers have found that we not only hold on because of our memories, but we also carry our ancestor's memories. It may sound crazy, but we carry *hand-me-down trauma*. Trauma from people we haven't ever met.

I've seen this trauma play out in a German friend of mine, Natasha, whose grandparents lived in Germany during World War II. Natasha is way too young to have lived through that war, yet she is riddled with guilt. She feels deep inside herself that she should have done something to stop the Nazis from persecuting and killing the Jews. But Natasha was not there or even alive during that time. This deep sense of not having done enough and feeling guilty because of her inaction is rooted deep into Natasha's being and affects her daily life.

Interesting, right? When I meet with clients like Natasha, who are deeply feeling something that they can't directly relate to in their own lives, I begin to question them about their ancestors.

One of the challenges in working with ancestral memories is that the sensations and/or feelings that are currently coming up could be resonating from an ancestor who lived so long ago that the stories of what occurred have died away from the family line. So, unlike Natasha, there may be no way to directly connect past trauma to the present feeling.

The low-back is caught in the middle of all of these memories, physical holds, emotional responses, mental beliefs, blocked energy pathways, traumas, and spiritual challenges. Based on that understanding, it's a wonder that everyone doesn't suffer from low-back pain.

I found on my journey out of low-back pain that I had to honor my whole body. As I worked on my physical body, it was necessary to release the emotions, beliefs, reactions, memories, and thoughts held in the tight blockages throughout my body.

To understand this, I studied the human body as a whole and where we hold certain emotions, beliefs, memories, and thoughts in the physical body. I had to learn how to locate them, then let them go.

I found that the process was like unwinding puppet strings that had gotten tangled up. I had to patiently untie the knots of tension and face my thoughts, memories, beliefs, emotions, and physical limitations in order to lengthen the strings (fascia and muscle) that needed to be long, and to strengthen or shorten the strings (fascia and muscle) that needed to be strong.

Okay, after all that complexity, I will attempt to simplify things. There are only four main causes of low-back pain. Let's dive into those right now!

Chapter 2 - The Four Roots of Low-Back Pain

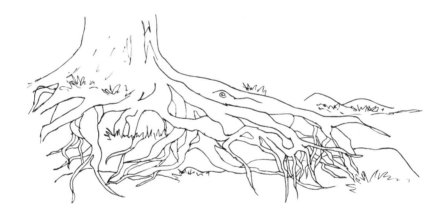

Tree
teach me roots
teach me the hidden why
Norman Crane

We'll begin by focusing on the most concrete and easily-assessable part of ourselves, the physical body. We are all made up of skin, bones, fascia, muscles, nerves, blood vessels, organs, joints, fluids, waste products, endorphins, chemicals, fat, hormones, energy, tissue, cells, and atoms.

To our physical bodies, we add emotions. We feel anxiety, fear, depression, sorrow, grief, anger, frustration, overwhelm, pessimism, optimism, hope, faith, trust, happiness, and joy. And these are just a few of the many emotions we feel at any given moment.

To our physical and emotional bodies, we add our brains and mental states; engaged, critical thinking, remembering, and autopilot.

And on top of all that…our spirituality. I like this definition of spirit: a sense of connection with others, a sense of life, and a relationship with a transcendent force.

Whoa, we are a complex miracle.

I will attempt to make our miraculous complex system as simple as possible. Luckily, I've found through my years of study that there are only four main root causes of low-back pain.

They are anger, control, fear, and stress.

We'll take them one by one and connect them physically, mentally, emotionally, energetically, and spiritually.

ANGER

Anger is a powerful emotion that gives us the energy to move and create change. When we can't handle something that causes us to react in rage or shut down, we store the unprocessed anger in our inner legs, in a muscle called the gracilis.

This gracilis muscle runs from the groin to the inside of the knee. Its purpose is to stabilize the pelvis. When this muscle gets filled with unprocessed anger, it no longer functions healthily. It gets stuck, tight, and often weak.

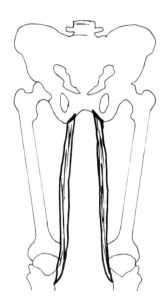

When the gracilis loses its ability to open and close freely as we move around on this earth, it no longer stabilizes the pelvis but causes it to become stuck, torqued, twisted, or too hypermobile, taking the impact of every move we make with our feet and our legs right in the sacral lumbar area.

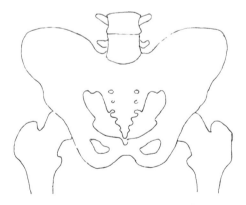

Pelvic stability is essential to a healthy low-back. Instability in the pelvic bowl can cause the pelvis to jam or twist and torque with every move. Over time, this can lead to a diagnosis of sacroiliac (SI) joint issues and/or lumbar vertebrae compression, leading to herniated discs, bulging discs, and degenerative disc disease.

The instability of the pelvis can cause sciatica, as the sacrum has holes that run down its sides for the nerves of the lower body to thread through. All these nerves come together in a large bundle called the sciatic nerve. When the sacrum is thrown off-center, the sciatic nerve can become pinched or impinged.

What can you do to stabilize the pelvic bowl? Open, release and strengthen the gracilis muscle to get it functioning again as you consciously release your anger with each out-breath.

Don't worry, I'll show you exactly how to diagnose tight gracilis muscles in your body and how to open, release and strengthen them step by step.

CONTROL

I like this definition of control: wanting something to be different than it is. Our brains don't know the difference between wanting something to be different and trying to control something so it will be different.

When we respond to something, whether it's outside of us or inside of us, with the thought that we want it to be different, we tighten our piriformis muscle. This muscle is found deep in our glutes and is where the phrase "tight ass" comes from.

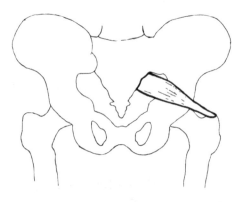

When the piriformis grabs, it can squeeze the sciatic nerve, which runs through the piriformis – or in some cases, right alongside the piriformis, which can cause sciatica.

The piriformis also attaches to the sacrum and the great trochanter (leg bone). When the piriformis is tight, it can pull the sacrum out of alignment and at the same time force the head of the femur (lesser trochanter) into the hip socket. This can cause hip pain or, in severe holds, ultimately lead to hip replacement as the head of the femur and the hip bone push toward one another until they are bone on bone.

Also, the squeeze of the piriformis can cause the sacrum to get stuck in an upward direction, which can cause the sacrum to jam into the low-back vertebrae. Again, this can lead to the diagnosis of sacroiliac (SI) joint issues and/or lumbar vertebrae compression, leading to herniated discs, bulging discs, and degenerative disc disease.

What can you do to release the piriformis? Open it as you consciously breathe out control and breathe in acceptance of all that is going on inside and outside of you.

Yes, I'll show you exactly how to diagnose tight piriformis muscles in your body and what to do to open and release them step by step.

FEAR

All mammals have fear muscles. They are built to help us to curl into a ball to protect our soft underbelly when we are at the mercy of a bear, lion, or other predators. They pull us into ourselves when we are afraid and feel like we need protection.

These fear muscles are found in the front of our bodies. They are the iliopsoas and quadriceps.

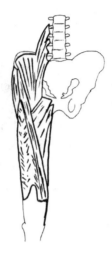

These muscles cause low-back pain by contracting in response to fear and often staying contracted after the fearful event has passed. Such contractions (after the danger has passed but the body is still tense) will produce anxiety.

When these muscles contract, they push the sacrum (the bottom of the spine) up into the lumbar vertebrae (lower back vertebrae), causing compression of the low-back vertebrae and contracting the low-back muscles, quadratus lumborum, and the erector spinea. When this contraction is severe it is called lordosis or swayback.

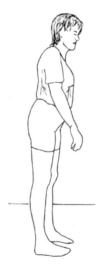

This contraction can lead to diagnoses such as herniated discs, bulging discs, slipped discs, degenerative disc disease, and stenosis. It can also be a cause of sciatica and other nerve issues down into the legs by compressing nerves between the vertebrae.

What can you do to take this compression off your low-back? Open and release your iliopsoas and quadriceps as you consciously breathe out fear.

And yes, I'll show you exactly how to diagnose tight iliopsoas and quad muscles in your body and how to open and release them step by step.

STRESS

Dr. John Sarno from New York University called low-back pain the *stress alarm bell* because whatever is going on in the upper body and/ or the lower body pulls on the low-back. For this reason, whenever my low-back hurts, I stop and ask myself, "What's bothering me?"

Many of you have chronic low-back pain that hurts every day. I experienced chronic low-back pain every single day for fifteen years, so I understand this misery. When I realized that my low-back was alerting me to how stressed out I was...I began to ask myself, "What am I holding on to that is causing me to be stressed out?" Over time, I began to figure it out.

When you stress out, your low-back contracts, which prevents the abdominals from working as your center core. When that happens, your belly weakens and protrudes forward, and your low-back has to do all the work for your abs, causing low-back tension and pain.

What can you do to let go of stress and release the contractions in the low-back? Relax, of course: open your iliopsoas, quads, piriformis, quadratus lumborum, and gracilis muscles and breathe out stress. Once you've released stress and have lengthened the low-back, you can begin the work of strengthening your core.

We'll get there! I'll show you exactly how to release your iliopsoas, quads, piriformis, quadratus lumborum, and gracilis muscles and how to let go of stress soon, but for now...We're going to dive into assessing your low-back.

Chapter 3 – Low-Back Pain Self-Assessment

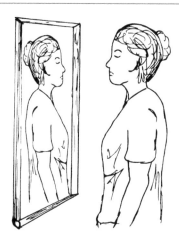

"Your visions will become clear only when you can look into your own heart. Who looks outside, dreams; who looks inside, awakes."
— **C.G. Jung**

Most of us with low-back pain have spent lots of time and money going to doctors, chiropractors, physical therapists, massage therapists, acupuncturists – anyone we heard about or read about, hoping to gain an understanding of what is causing our low-back pain and ultimately what we can do to release the pain.

In my fifteen-year quest to end my low-back pain, I got very little helpful information from traditional medicine. I've sat with thousands of people who've spent so much time and money attempting to get answers and a cure for their back pain, with little or nothing to show for it.

When I meet with a client for the first time they almost always say to me, *"No one but you has looked at my whole body to see what is going on with my low-back."*

I don't know why this is, but I believe the medical community doesn't know what to do with low-back pain sufferers.

I didn't give up. I kept seeking answers and experimenting with the things I learned. As a result, I have come up with a simple way to do a low-back self-assessment. I created it to help you understand what is causing your low-back pain.

A Pain-Free Low-Back Story

I met Jess after she'd been suffering from low-back pain for twenty years. She'd tried everything the medical community recommended and because she's a massage therapist, she also got lots and lots of therapeutic massages. None of the treatments worked. The traditional medical community was out of options and gave up on her. Jess almost gave up on herself as well.

Fortunately, Jess heard about my work. We met, I assessed her low-back, and she began to do the work outlined in this book.

Here's what Jess has to say now. *"The doctors had given up on me and told me that I'd have to live with my low-back pain. Michelle told me not to give up when she assessed my low-back.*

No doctor had ever really looked at All Of Me. I'm so glad she saw what was going on with my low-back. I'm so happy I followed her suggestions because I'm out of low-back pain.

I can even shovel snow for two hours without my low-back hurting! If my low-back pain starts to come back, I know exactly what to do to get right back out of the pain. After living with low-back pain for twenty years, I'm so relieved."

A couple of things before you begin:

- Wear something tight-fitting and light-colored.
- You'll need to have a full-length mirror.

- Be barefoot.
- Keep an open mind.
- Follow the instructions step-by-step.
- Smile, this is your first step out of low-back pain.

A Simple low-back Self-Assessment

Examine Your Body in a Full-Length Mirror

ANGER –

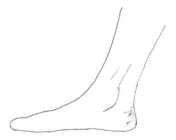

Look at the arches of your feet. Are they collapsing in? This is called flat feet and is caused by weak gracilis (inner leg) muscles. The inner leg is the pelvic stabilizer and the gracilis muscle has to be active to keep the pelvis in alignment.

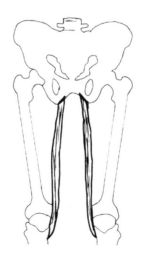

When the gracilis is tight and weak, you are holding on to anger. When the pelvis goes out of alignment, it can cause hyper-mobility in the low-back, which can lead to twists and torques in the low-back and can cause degenerative disc disease, herniated discs, slipped discs, bulging discs, and SI Joint Issues.

You may be aware of feeling angry, having outbursts of side-ways anger or rage, and experiencing generalized frustration and resentment.

ANSWER THESE QUESTIONS:

1. Are the arches in your feet collapsed causing flat feet?
2. What are you angry about?

CONTROL

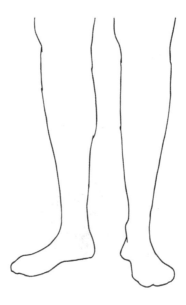

Look down at your feet and notice the direction your feet point. If they duck out, you have tight piriformis muscles located deep in the glutes.

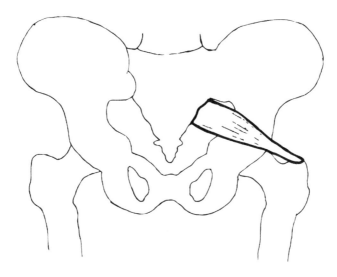

A tight piriformis muscle means you are wanting to control something that you wish was different than it is.

Check to see if one foot is pulled over more than another. This means you have a tighter piriformis on one side. The right foot being pulled to the right means that you are controlling others. The left foot being pulled to the left means you are controlling yourself.

The desire to control can cause feelings of anger, fear, and depression. The contraction of the piriformis muscle causes the sacrum to be stuck, leading to degenerative disc disease, herniated discs, slipped discs, bulging discs, and SI Joint Issues.

Answer these questions:

1. Do your feet duck out?
2. Does one foot duck out more than the other? The right foot or the left foot?
3. What do you want to be different right now?

FEAR –

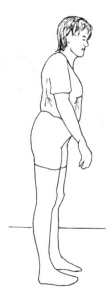

Turn to your side to look at your pelvic bowl. Is the back part of your pelvic bowl (sacrum) lifting up, and do your hip bones in the front fall down and forward? Does your belly bulge out and hang down? This means your illopsoas muscles in the front of your body are tight. The iliopsoas is the fear muscle.

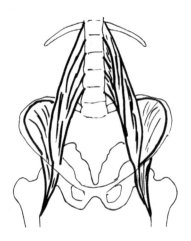

This posture says you are in fear, and this held fear is causing your sacrum to jam into your low-back vertebrae (L5-1). This can cause degenerative disc disease, herniated discs, slipped discs, bulging discs, SI Joint issues, sciatica, and low-back pain from compression of the quadratus lumborum (QL) muscles.

You may be aware of feeling anxious, or maybe you've even been diagnosed with an anxiety disorder.

Answer these questions:

1. Does your sacrum lift up into your low-back?
2. Do your hip bones in the front of your pelvis dip down?
3. Is your belly hanging out and down?
4. What are you afraid of?

STRESS

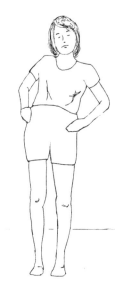

Place your hands on your hips. Is one hip lifting up on one side more than the other? This is caused by a tight quadratus lumborum (QL), the stress muscle.

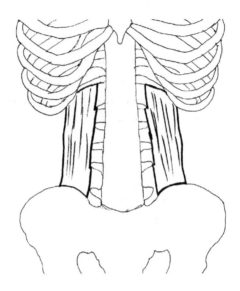

If the right hip is lifting, the outer world is stressing you out. If the left hip is lifting, your inner world of feelings, intuition and inner knowings are stressing you. Stress is a mixture of fear, anger, and the desire to control.

This compression on one side of your low-back can cause degenerative disc disease, herniated discs, slipped discs, bulging discs, sciatica, and SI joint issues.

You may be feeling anxious, angry, or depressed.

Answer these questions:

1. Is your right or left hip lifting?
2. What is stressing you out right now?

A Low-Back Pain Relief Story –
I began working with Holly right after she lost her life partner. Her low-back pain and sciatica were so bad that she couldn't even make it up the stairs to sleep in her bed.

Holly understood after her low-back assessment that she had all the issues that cause low-back pain: fear, stress, loss of control, and anger. She didn't know how she was going to go on after losing her best friend and partner.

After only a few weeks of working together Holly said, "*Michelle has saved my life. I was hanging on emotionally so hard and was in such severe low-back pain that painkillers did nothing for me. But now my low-back pain is receding. I can walk upstairs to sleep again, and I feel hopeful about my future.*"

Part II: The Cause Of Low-Back Pain - Digging Deeper

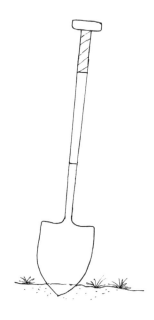

" I don't know anything, but I do know that everything is interesting if you go into it deeply enough." – Richard Feynman

Chapter 4 – What is Fascia?

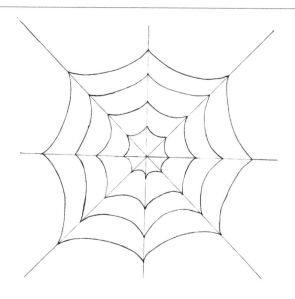

I am an imperfect sculpture
Of life' beautiful scars
Guarded by spiderweb curtains
Tammy M. Darby

About thirteen years into my yoga practice (after the terrible night on the floor when I found the golf ball), I began to use ball-rolling to release fascia. I didn't really understand fully what I was doing, but as soon as I added ball work to my movement practice, my low-back pain reduced, I could go deeper into poses, my posture improved, and I felt better overall.

I came to realize that working on the fascia was a key to releasing my low-back pain. I didn't know anything about fascia, so I decided to dive deep into the study of fascia with Tom Myers, the author of *Anatomy Trains*. What I found was fascinating!! So, I'm going to share the most important parts of this incredible fascia system with you.

"Fascia is the missing element in the movement/stability equation," says Tom Myers. *"While anatomy lists around 600 separate muscles, it is more accurate to say that there is one muscle poured into six hundred pockets of the fascial webbing. The 'illusion' of separate muscles is created by the anatomist's scalpel, dividing tissues along the planes of fascia. This reductive process should not blind us to the reality of the unifying whole."*

So fascia is a whole interconnected system. And here's something that will really blow your mind: your fascia has memory and awareness!

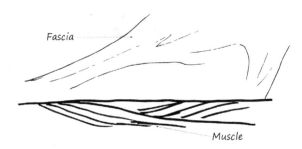

Fascia

Muscle

According to cardiologist Dr. Bruno Bordoni, who wrote the article "The Awareness of the Fascial System," *"A fascial cell has not only memory but also the awareness of the mechanometabolic information it feels, and it has the anticipatory predisposition in preparing itself for alteration of its natural environment."*

Yes, you read that right, your fascia feels and remembers. It also impacts you emotionally. Dr. Bruno Bordini goes on to state in his article "Anatomy Fascia," *"The fascial unity influences not only movement but also emotions. A dysfunction of the fascial system that is perpetuated in every-day movements can cause an emotional alteration of the person. This emotional alteration could be established originating from constant myofascial non-physiological afferents, which would bring the emotional state and the myofascial pathology to the same level. In fact, the position of the body stimulates areas of emotionality, and the presence of myofascial alterations leads to postural alterations."*

But wait, there's even more. According to the article "The Structure That Carries Consciousness" by Marisa Chadbourne, LNT, JFB Myofascial Therapist. *"Many scientists and bodywork therapists believe consciousness is tangible and can be touched. The fascial system, a super network of connective tissue, is the physical doorway we can use to enter into consciousness. Fascia permeates our entire being three dimensionally, uninterrupted from head to toe—through every organ, muscle and bone, precisely infusing into each and every cell. Within this extraordinary system lies a network of communication that is comparable to the operating system of a computer. The brain acts like the hard drive as it signals our bodies to move, organs to function, and holds astounding intelligence all on its own."*

Are you getting this?? Your fascia contracts, releases, feels, remembers, and anticipates...which impacts your posture and the way you move. It's your most active sensory organ. It can contract independently of the muscles it encases, and it responds to stress without your conscious command. It is described above as *the carrier of your consciousness.*

This is huge!

It means that your fascia is impacting all your movements and your emotions, all the time.

So, exactly what is fascia?

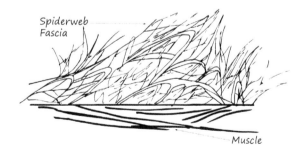

Spiderweb Fascia

Muscle

According to James F. Barnes, PT, *"Fascia is a specialized system of the body that has an appearance similar to a spider's web or a sweater. Fascia is very densely woven, covering and interpenetrating every muscle, bone, nerve, artery, and vein, as well as all of our internal organs, including the heart, lungs, brain, and spinal cord. The most interesting aspect of the fascial system is that it is not just a system of separate coverings. It is actually one continuous structure that exists from head to toe without interruption. In this way, you can begin to see that each part of the entire body is connected to every other part by the fascia, like the yarn in a sweater."*

Everything that happens to you affects the fascia. Everything: all thoughts, actions, traumas, inflammatory responses, accidents, injuries, and surgical procedures. Life itself can basically create myofascial restrictions that may produce pressure on pain-sensitive structures that do not show up in many of the standard low-back pain tests, such as X-rays, MRIs, and CAT scans. This leads to a high percentage of people suffering from low-back pain, tension, and lack of motion who may be having fascial problems but are not diagnosed because they show no symptoms on traditional tests.

Fascia plays an important role in the support and function of our bodies since it surrounds and attaches to all structures. In its normal, healthy state, the fascia is relaxed, soft, and wavy. It can stretch and move without restriction.

When one experiences physical trauma, emotional trauma, scarring, or inflammation, however, the fascia loses its pliability. It becomes tight, restricted, and a source of tension for the rest of the body.

Trauma, such as a fall, car accident, whiplash, surgery, or just habitual poor posture and repetitive stress injuries have cumulative effects on the entire body. The changes trauma causes in the fascial system influence the comfort and function of the body. Fascial restrictions can create excessive pressure causing all kinds of symptoms, including low-back pain or restriction of motion.

Fascial restrictions affect our flexibility and stability and are a key factor in our ability to withstand stress and perform daily activities.

Try this…

From *Understanding your Fascia* by Julia Lucus — "*Grab hold of the collar of your shirt and give it a little tug. Your whole shirt responds, right? Your collar pulls into the back of your neck. The tail of your shirt inches up the small of your back. Your sleeves move up your forearms. Then it falls back into place. That's a bit like fascia. It fits like a giant, body-hugging T-shirt over your whole body, from the top of your head to the tips of your toes and crisscrossing back and forth and through and back again. You can't move just one piece of it, and you can't make a move without bringing it along.*

Fascinating, right? So pull the front collar of your shirt again and think about pulling it forward and holding it for an eight-hour workday, just like you sit hunched over your computer or desk at work. How about pulling and releasing your pant legs about two thousand times? That's like going for a twenty-minute run.

If you did this to your clothes, your clothes would be pretty messed up. But fascia has self-healing properties and is a very tough substance. When fascia is healthy it is very flexible, allowing you to move, stretch, and contract; it then returns to its smooth resting state. Over time the fascia fibers can thicken and gum up as the fascia responds to stress and trauma. Poor posture, making repetitive movements, and living a sedentary lifestyle can cause a decrease in the fascia's flexibility. Scars can form when stuck fascia is asked to move and cannot.

Seems like this could be problematic, but every bit of damage your fascia endures can be healed. And you can learn to take care of your fascia to avoid future issues.

How to Take Care of Your Fascia

1. **Create a Daily Movement Practice that you do first thing every morning.** Including yoga stretching, strengthening, and most importantly…

2. **Include ball-rolling in your Daily Movement Practice.** Roll different-sized balls (like lacrosse, softball-sized, tennis, and golf balls) back and forth and side to side to break up the tension in your fascia. Remember, fascia can withstand up

to two thousand pounds of pressure, so you're not going to force your body open. Be gentle and move slowly.

3. **Learn to breathe fully and deeply from your diaphragm.** Your breath will massage and loosen your fascia from the inside out.

4. **Drink lots of water every day!** Your body is about sixty percent water for a reason — it operates better when lubricated! So keep your water levels high to keep your fascia and whole body functioning well.

5. **Learn to let go and allow your body to hang out and rest.** In yoga, there is a saying that the rest is as important as the movement. Make resting as important as moving in your life.

6. **Listen to your body.** When it says to stop doing whatever you're doing, don't keep pushing it — stop. Our culture is currently out of balance and is more masculine than feminine, which encourages all of us to overdo nearly every life activity, such as working, exercising, and eating. It's time to bring your body into a balance between doing and being.

A Low-Back Pain Relief Story –

By the time Wendy's orthopedic surgeon told her that the only way to possibly release her low-back pain was to undergo surgery, she'd had nine jaw surgeries and didn't want to go under the knife ever again. So Wendy started going to a pain clinic to try to ease her low-back pain. She got prescriptions but very little relief.

That's when Wendy found me. I assessed her body and noticed that she had tight piriformis (control) muscles, tight iliopsoas (fear) muscles, and a sacroiliac (SI) joint that went out on her right side.

I gave Wendy her practice: to release her piriformis and iliopsoas muscles. I showed her how to put her SI joint back in place. Wendy soon became pain-free and got back to taking the daily walks with her dogs that she so loved.

Wendy says, *"I start every day with myofascial release ball work and I no longer go to the pain clinic, get injections, nerve blocks or take pain pills. I am pain-free and I am so grateful!"*

Chapter 5 – Fascia + Muscle Move Bone

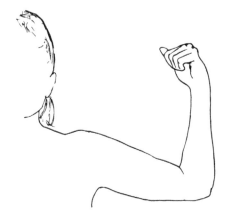

Contemporary therapists need to think "outside the box" of this isolated muscle concept. – Tom Myers, *Anatomy Trains*

Your fascia is like a baggie, and inside the baggie is the muscle, which is like hamburger meat. When you move the baggie the hamburger meat moves, just like when you move the fascia, the muscle moves. When the fascia is pulled, the muscle is also pulled, often tightening it into a contraction. That contraction will move the nearby bones.

For example, when someone has scoliosis, you can look at their spine and see how the tightness on the right side of the low-back spine is pulling the lumbar spine to the right.

This pulling is happening all over your body. Wherever you carry tension, the fascia is pulling, the muscle is contracting, and the muscle is moving the bones out of alignment.

Unfortunately, according to KidsHealth Medical Experts, *Muscles can pull bones, but they can't push them back to their original position.*

Bottom line: when your fascia tells a muscle to contract, it does and will hold that muscle in a contraction for as long as the brain tells it to stay contracted. The muscle pressure from the contraction will pull the nearby bones and joints out of alignment.

In the low-back, this means: The muscle contractions in the gracilis muscles located in the inner legs will destabilize the pelvic bowl, allowing the sacrum and hips to move in ways that they weren't designed to move. This hypermobility can cause the sacroiliac (SI) joints, hip joints, and lumbar vertebrae to move out of alignment, which can cause SI Joint problems, hip challenges, twists and torques in the pelvic bowl, degenerative disc disease, herniated discs, bulging discs, stenosis, and sciatica.

The chronic contraction of the iliopsoas muscles, located from the inside of your hip bone and down into the crease at the top of your leg (inguinal crease), can cause the sacral bone to shove up into the lumbar vertebrae, causing compression which can lead to degenerative disc disease, herniated discs, bulging discs, stenosis, and sciatica.

Also, the piriformis muscle, located under the gluteus muscles in the butt cheeks, when chronically contracted can press into the sacrum, locking it in place. This can cause a jarring of the lumbar vertebrae, which can create SI Joint problems, hip challenges, twists and torques in the pelvic bowl, degenerative disc disease, herniated discs, bulging discs, stenosis, and sciatica.

And then, the quadratus lumborum muscle, located in the low-back, when held in place by a contraction will pull the lumbar spine, sacrum, and hip joints out of alignment. This can cause herniated discs, bulging discs, sacrum issues, and hip joint challenges.

In summary, your fascia has brain cells in it which tell specific muscles to contract. The muscle contracts, which over time moves the nearby bones and joints out of alignment, causing structural issues that can cause pain. When this happens in the inner legs, butt cheeks, front of the hips, and the low-back area we experience low-back pain!

A Pain-Free Low-Back Story –

When I met Tina she was getting ready for her son's wedding but was very worried because she could barely walk because of her low-back pain and sciatica that was radiating into her butt cheek and down her leg.

Tina wanted desperately to dance at her son's wedding and said, *I was attracted to talk to Michelle because I wanted to get out of low-back pain as quickly as possible to enjoy my son's wedding to the fullest. I was worried, I could barely stand and walk much less dance the night away. I began doing the work Michelle told me to do and I'm literally living with a ball in my butt cheek now. The myofascial release ball work allowed me to dance at my son's wedding and it's allowing my low-back pain to recede.*

Now, let's dive deeper into why the brain tells these muscles to contract by learning a bit about the energy pathways of the body.

Chapter 6 – You Are An Energy Body

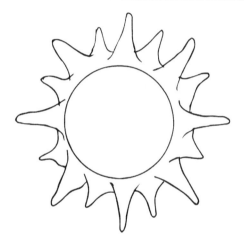

"Be your own energy drink."
— Hiral Nagda

Your body was built to allow energy and fluids to flow freely in and out of it. But something happens along the way and you begin to block the flow, just like a river when a big log falls in and dams up the flow of water.

I began to introduce the energy maps of the body when I shared that the gracilis muscles hold unprocessed anger, the iliopsoas muscles are the fear muscles, the piriformis muscles are the control muscles, and the quadratus lumborum muscles are the stress muscles.

You can think of anger, fear, control, and stress as the logs that dam up your energy flow.

We are going to explore how you are built energetically so that you can have a deeper understanding of why your brain contracts certain muscles and holds them in a chronic contraction, causing a log jam in the energy flow of your body.

Where does this energy body information come from? Let's look back into our past. Yes, our ancestors from the east were the first to understand that we have energy running through our bodies, and they were the first people to map it out. Awareness of this ancient Eastern energy information has influenced us throughout history, all the way up to our system of modern Western medicine.

These are the seven energy systems I have studied and regularly address to understand the energy body as a whole. These seven energy systems include:

- Meridians, which are energy pathways of the body mapped out in Chinese medicine.
- Chakras, which means "wheels," refers to energy points in the body. They are thought to be spinning discs of energy that should stay "open" and aligned, as they correspond to bundles of nerves, major organs, and areas of our energetic body that affect our emotional and physical well-being. They come from the Vedas in India. (My Chakra teacher is Christine Page, MD. I met her when I was working for Presbyterian Hospital in Dallas, TX as a yoga therapist. She was teaching physicians about the energy system of the body.)
- Aura is a part of the chakra system and is thought to be a luminous body that surrounds your physical one.
- Reiki comes from the Japanese words "rei," meaning universal, and "ki," which means vital life force energy that flows through all living things. Some practitioners describe reiki as acupuncture without needles.

- The body's three main energy systems: ATP-PC, Glycolytic, and Oxidative were classified by modern western science and are based on how we use food to fuel our bodies.
- The Basic Grid, Celtic Weave, Five Rhythms, Triple Warmer, Radiant Circuits, and the Electrics are from Donna Eden's Energy Medicine.
- Hands of light, Barbara Brennan's healing modality. She is a former NASA Physicist.

I have studied this vast array of energy systems and will break down the energy maps of the body as simply as possible.

First of all, you are a human and a spirit. Human Energy flows throughout the bottom portion of your body, from the navel on down. The energy is heavy and contains the need to root and create. It also holds the lower emotions of depression, fear, sorrow, anger, frustration, overwhelm, and pessimism.

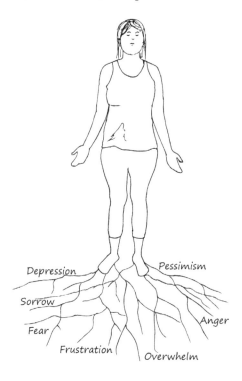

The middle of your body is where your human meets your spirit and contains lighter energy that wants to power you to move and fulfill your purpose. It holds the energy of pessimistic optimism.

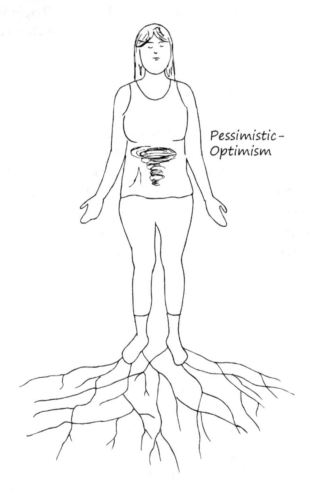

Pessimistic-Optimism

At the top of your body, from your heart all the way up to over your head, runs spirit energy. This is light energy that wants to move up to love, speak your heart's truth, see your reality, and connect to the greater energy in all. It holds the energy of optimism, faith, hope, trust, happiness, and joy.

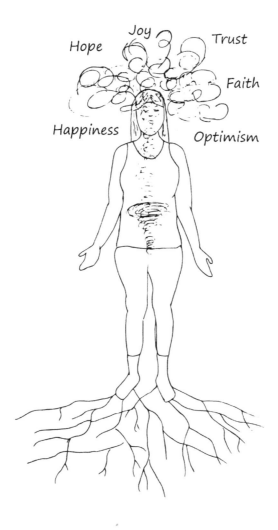

You are also masculine and feminine energy combined. Your masculine energy runs on the right side of your body. This is your outer-world-focused doer, thinker, and analyzer. It represents your sympathetic nervous system.

Your feminine energy lies on the left side of your body and is your inner-world-focused being, feeler, and intuitive. It represents your parasympathetic nervous system.

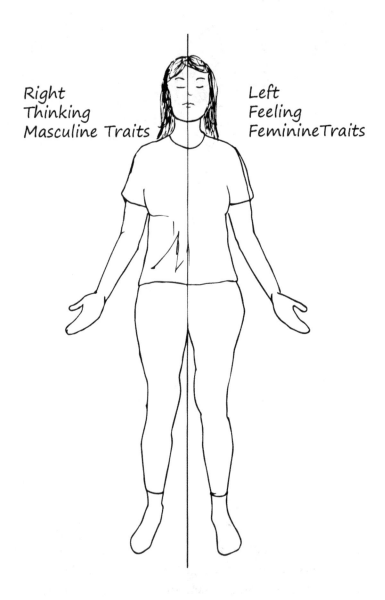

Right
Thinking
Masculine Traits

Left
Feeling
FeminineTraits

You also have a front of the body which is known as the light side of the body. The back is the unknown or the shadow side of the body.

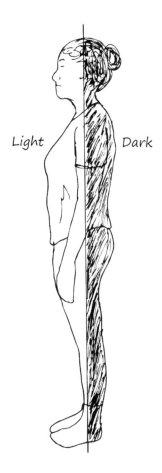

Light   Dark

I know this may be new information and can seem complicated, but I will make everything crystal clear as we go along.

A Pain-Free Low-Back Story –
Beth was in low-back pain and nothing she did made it better. She couldn't drive any distance without her low-back flaring up. That's when she reached out to me. I assessed her posture and found that the left (feminine) side of her body was noticeably tighter than her right (masculine) side.

Beth shared how in her household growing up, her mother didn't allow feelings. Beth's mom had grown up with a very needy mother (Beth's grandmother) and because of this Beth's mom attributed feelings to neediness. As a result, Beth learned at a very young age not to share her feelings – until she began to have chronic low-back pain.

Beth started her Pain-Free Low-Back Posture Daily Practice with the awareness of opening up to the feminine feeling side of her body and feeling her emotions. Beth's low-back pain decreased so much that within a few short days she took her elderly parents for two long car rides to enjoy the last of the summer weather.

Beth says *I can't believe it. I wish I'd reached out to Michelle much sooner. I had no idea I could feel this good this fast!*

Chapter 7 - Posture of Pain

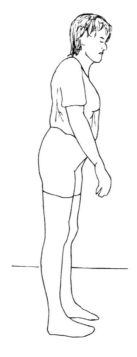

Pain

pain surrounds you day to day
nothing helps it go away
pain in muscles pain in joints
pain so bad in trigger points.

Leticia Starkey

Those of us with low-back pain live in a posture of pain without even being aware of it. In the fifteen years I suffered from chronic low-back pain, I bounced from physical therapists, doctors, and chiropractors to massage therapists, yoga therapists, and psychotherapists. No one – and I mean not one of the practitioners I sought out to help me with my low-back pain – looked at my posture.

NOT ONE.

The thousands of people I've helped out of low-back pain tell me, *"You are the first person to just really look at my body."*

What is up with that?

Traditional medicine practitioners like to do MRIs, CAT Scans, and X-rays…but looking at a patient, really assessing them, and talking to them…well, that just doesn't happen. And the crazy thing is that if you just look at someone experiencing low-back pain, their body posture tells their pain story.

It takes me about five minutes of looking at a new client to know exactly what is causing their low-back pain. The fascia and muscle contractions show up when you look at a person standing up.

They typically, like me, have one or more of these postural issues:

- A sacrum that pushes up into their lumbar vertebrae because the iliopsoas muscles in the front of their body are tight.
- A hip that is pulled forward because the iliopsoas muscle on one side is tighter.
- A hip that is higher on one side than the other because of a tighter quadratus lumborum.
- Feet that duck out, indicating tight piriformis muscles in their butt cheeks. which causes a further jam into the lumbar vertebrae.
- A belly that protrudes forward because they are not using their abdominals for core strength but rather the quadratus lumborum muscles in the low-back.

Because of the posture of low-back pain, they may have sacrums that have slipped out, nerves that are pinched, a narrowing of the bony openings within the spine called stenosis, herniated discs, bulging discs, slipped discs, degenerative disc disease, and arthritis.

Their body is literally screaming at them about the fear, anger, control, or stress held deep inside.

Most people who have a screaming low-back and at least one of these diagnoses have tried so many things to stop the pain, and nothing works. I'm encouraging those of you who feel you've tried everything, don't give up. You are about to learn how to get yourself out of your low-back pain!

You can do it. You just need to know how.

A Pain-Free Low-Back Story –
Mitch was working hard in his backyard when suddenly his back went out. He was in excruciating pain. His body was bent forward at the hips and he shuffled as he walked. Mitch contacted me after trying painkillers for a week with no reduction in his pain.

I assessed Mitch's back and could see that his iliopsoas (fear) muscles were super-contracted. I gave Mitch a daily practice of myofascial release ball work and stretching of the iliopsoas muscle. This is what Mitch said two weeks later. *I'm now out of low-back pain! It's baffling to me that I could get into so much pain, and not be able to get out of it. When I understood what was causing it and began to work on it, my low-back pain faded away. I will keep doing my low-back practice to stay out of pain.*

So, let's get started and do what Mitch did to get out of low-back pain!

Part III: The Cure – Your Daily Practice

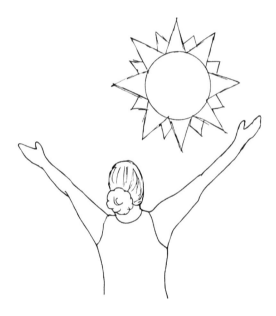

"The question is not how to get cured, but how to live." — Joseph Conrad

Chapter 8 - The Way Out of Low-Back Pain

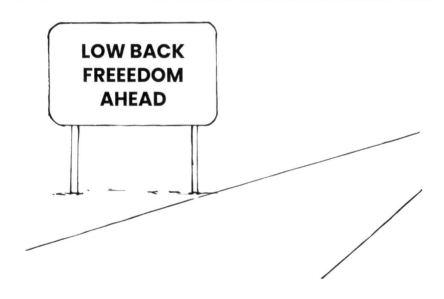

"When there's no way out, you just follow the way in front of you."
— Stephen Mitchell

I've listed below the steps to take and the tools you need to work your way out of back pain.

A Daily Practice – The first and most important step to low-back pain relief is to have a daily practice that addresses the whole body and releases it from chronic holding patterns, emotional and mental blocks, and spiritual challenges. Commit to a daily practice that allows the body to open and flow with life instead of pushing against it.

Breathwork – The breath is the healer from the inside out. There is one breathing method that I've found to be the most helpful. I call it the *Haaaa* Breath, and it is very simple.

You just breathe in through your nose and down into your lungs, feeling your belly rise up and the lungs expand as you breathe in. This means you are using your diaphragm.

Breathe out of your mouth saying, *"Haaaa"* as the air leaves your lungs and your belly draws back toward your spine.

Haaaa is the energy vibration of the heart – as in aloha, the Hawaiian way of greeting one another. Aloha means the breath of love. So as you do the *Haaaa* Breath, you are breathing out fear, anger, stress, control, and breathing in love.

Try it right now!

Take a deep breath in and as you breathe out say, "*Haaaa*", and visualize fear leaving your body. Take three more *Haaaa* Breaths and notice how you feel.

Myofascial Release Ball Work – Most of us can't afford a myofascial release massage therapist to come to the house every day to release our fascia. So learning how to release your fascia by massaging with balls of various sizes is key to low-back pain relief.

It is important to repeatedly massage the fascia that is holding a muscle in a contraction. The goal is to release the fascia, rather than just sitting on a knot of tension. So, always stay in continual motion, going back and forth or up and down with the ball.

It was only when I started using the balls to roll out my fascia every day that my low-back finally began to release its chronically held pain.

Stretching – Stretching the muscles that you've released with the myofascial ball work is the next important step in a Pain-Free

Low-Back Daily Practice. Once you are in a stretch, it is important to work your way up to holding each pose for two minutes, as it has been proven that holding a pose for ninety seconds or more makes the mind-body connection. You must give the opening that you create in a pose time to get the message to the brain that you really want to let go.

If you rapidly move from pose to pose, that mind-body connection isn't established, and the body will stay stuck in its holding pattern.

Strengthening – As your body opens with ball work, breath work, and stretching, it is vital to practice a Pain-Free Low-Back Posture, so that the bones fall back into their anatomically correct place from the release of the fascia and muscle holds.

Strengthening the muscles that need to be strengthened will keep the new posture in alignment and keep you feeling good as you get back to doing the things you love like hiking, swimming, walking, playing with your kids or grandkids, cooking, shopping, or whatever brings you joy!

Let go – That sounds much easier than it is. The things we need to let go of to free ourselves from our low-back pain are the very things we hold onto – so tightly that we've incorrectly and painfully postured our bodies to keep hanging on to them.

With this practice, you'll let go with each out-breath of "*Haaaa*". You'll release the anger gripping your inner legs. You'll let go of the fears that you may have held in your iliopsoas since childhood. You'll slowly unwind the grip of control, allowing your glutes and piriformis to soften. As you lengthen your quadratus lumborum to strengthen your belly, you'll unwind the stress alarm bell that may have been blaring for years in your low-back.

Movement Tools – It's time to go shopping. Listed below are all the tools you will need for the suggested ball work and movements in this book. You can purchase them from your local discount depart-ment store or order them online.

Yoga Mat
I prefer a lightweight one so that it's easy to move around.

Blanket
A beach towel or a lightweight couch throw.

Noodle Ball and Swimming Pool Noodle

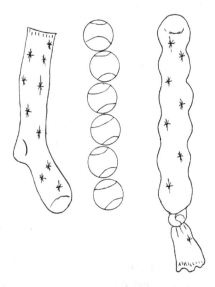

To make a Noodle Ball, take a knee-high sock and stuff six tennis balls into the sock. Push the balls towards the bottom of the sock and tie a knot at the last ball. Make sure the balls are snug and tight.

Some of you will find using the Noodle Ball too intense in the beginning. To get used to the Noodle Ball, you can get a swimming pool noodle and use that instead. Buy a regular-size swimming pool noodle and cut it to the width of your upper back.

Softball-sized Ball
A 3.5-inch massage ball or regular softball.

Yoga Strap
Any strap or belt will do. If you buy one, get the extra-long yoga strap.

Yoga Block
The light foam ones are good and super-easy to find these days.

Art Supplies
Gather old magazines that you can cut up, heavy art paper, cardboard, or index cards. If you like to draw, paint or crayon, pick up your favorite art tools. Scissors and glue are necessary items. Yes, you're going to get creative!

Chapter 9 - The Pain-Free Low-Back Posture

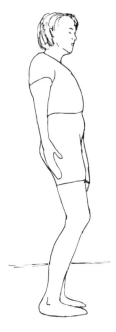

*"Our nonverbal behavior (including posture) gives away our
inner personality and reflects our inner attitude."*
— Cindy Ann Peterson

Every person with low-back pain has a posture that shows what
is creating the pain. As I said, I can find the trouble spot in less
than five minutes. The low-back pain posture not only shows

what is causing the physical pain but also shows the underlying emotional and mental pain.

The cure to releasing low-back pain is to learn to posture the physical body in a way that takes the pressure, tension, and pain off the low-back and out of the emotional and mental fields at the same time.

EVERYTHING I'm going to teach you from here on is all about creating your new Pain-Free Low-Back Posture.

I will begin by introducing you to the Pain-Free Low-Back Posture right now. I want you to try it, but remember, it's not going to be easy. I'll be here showing you how to build your new Pain-Free Low-Back Posture step-by-step.

PAIN-FREE LOW-BACK POSTURE STANDING –

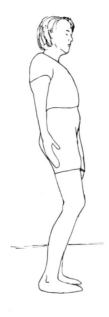

- Stand with your feet inner-hip width apart. I place my hands at the inside of my hip bones, point my fingertips down and look down, lining up my feet with my hips, knees, and ankles.
- Make sure your feet are lined up and facing straight ahead. No ducking out or pigeon-toeing in.

- Press into the outer edges of your heels as you lift and spread your toes.
- Create a soft bend to your knees.
- Slightly roll your inner legs in.
- Pat out your butt cheeks to make sure they are loose and free.
- Drop your tail and sacrum down as if just beginning to sit in a chair.
- Lift your hip bones up.
- Draw your ribs in and down which begins to work your abdominals.
- Roll your inner arms out.
- Squeeze your shoulder blades together and take them down toward your tail.
- Allow your head and neck to be loose and free.

As you try this, notice how the new Pain-Free Low-Back Posture feels. It will feel awkward at first because we are changing the way you've stood since childhood.

PAIN-FREE LOW-BACK POSTURE WALKING –

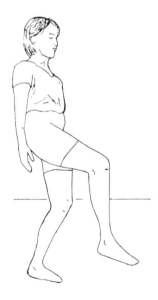

- Take the Pain-Free Low-Back Standing Posture detailed above.
- Sit back as if starting to sit in a chair.
- Walk with your legs in front of you and your upper body floating loose and free.

PAIN-FREE LOW-BACK POSTURE SITTING –

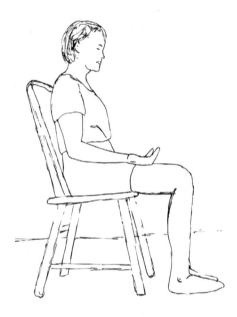

- Stand in front of a chair and take the Pain-Free Low-Back Standing Posture detailed above.
- Sit back as if sitting in the chair and keep going until you are actually sitting in the chair.
- As you sit, keep your tail down.
- Snap your ribs in and down.
- Roll your inner arms out, squeeze your shoulder blades together, and take them down toward your low-back.

Notice your challenges as you practice these new postures. Just observe. Don't get frustrated or give up. You've been walking, sitting, and standing the way you do for many, many years. It will take practice to make the new Pain-Free Low-Back Posture easy and comfortable.

A Pain-Free Low-Back Story –
Bob is a big strong man who loves to landscape, which means he's done some very heavy lifting over the years. Unfortunately, Bob is now in his seventies, and all that heavy lifting caused chronic low-back pain that was halting his landscaping passion.

When I met Bob, he was moving very cautiously and visibly wincing with every step he took. I assessed his posture and noticed a big pull of his piriformis (control) muscle. I suggested a practice he needed to do every day. He immediately began this daily practice, and this is what happened.

Bob stated in his own words, *I thought I'd never be able to pick up heavy rocks, cut down trees, and move soil ever again. But with the daily practice I learned from Michelle, I can get back into my yard and create my vision. I'm so very happy I found her because I was seeing a pain specialist who was giving me painkillers and injections and they were not doing a thing.*

Part III: The Cure – Create Your NEW Pain-Free Low-Back Posture

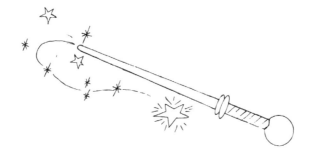

*"The great Way is easy,
yet people prefer the side paths.
Be aware when things are out of balance."*
— Lao Tzu, *Tao Te Ching*

A couple of notes to make your journey into your Pain-Free Low-Back Posture smooth and easy.

- Take this slowly so that you have time to process what is shifting for you. I would suggest doing the feet movement work and answering the questions on the first day, then moving on to the leg practice and questions the next day, then continuing up the body one area a day.

- Do what you can. If something is too challenging, don't do it and make a note in the book, as it was designed as a workbook.
- Make a note of the exercises and practices that have the greatest impact on you.
- Remember the *Haaaa* Breath. Use it while you do each practice.
- Your Full Pain-Free Low-Back Daily Practice will be outlined at the end of the book.
- Enjoy the journey. You are working your way out of low-back pain!

Chapter 10 - Release Your Feet, Legs, and Anger to Form a Strong Foundation

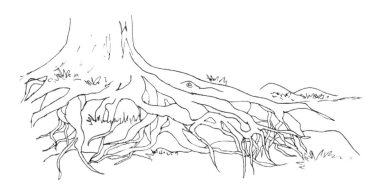

"If you know where you are from, it will be harder for people to stop you where you are going." — Matshona Dhliwayo

To create your Pain-Free Low-Back Posture Daily Practice, you must begin at your feet, the deepest root and the foundation of your body. You will learn to posture your feet and legs in a new way that supports your pelvic bowl and allows your sacrum to drop down as your hip bones lift up.

While you work to physically create a posture that releases low-back pain, you will also release anger and address your DNA, genetics, and childhood traumas.

Let's get started on this incredible journey into your foundation.

Your Feet Movement Practice

You'll need a yoga mat and a golf ball.

Ball Work – The Feet

Roll a Golf Ball on The Soles of Your Feet –

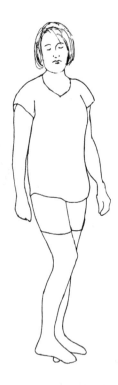

Stand on a golf ball and roll it around on the soles of your feet, feeling for knots of tension. Stay on the knots and breathe into your feet and out from your feet saying, *"Haaaa"* while you focus on who brought you into this life: your ancestors. Honor dad's ancestors as you roll on the bottom of your right foot. Honor your mom's ancestors as you roll on the bottom of your left foot.

Stretches – The Feet

Sit on Your Toes to Open Your Soles –

All Fours –

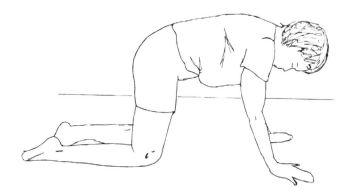

Come into a cat by bringing your knees under your hips and your hands under your shoulders on all fours. Bring your ribs up and in toward your pelvis, roll your inner arms out and squeeze your scapula together, keeping a long lower back. From there, you can move your head and neck around and circle your hips in both directions.

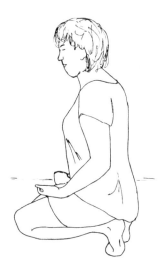

Tuck your toes under and begin to make circles with your hips. Go both directions and then sit back on your heels.

Walk your hands up to your knees. If your knees don't hurt, keep walking your hands up your thighs until you are sitting up straight.

Make sure your little toe is being sat on. Take your tail down, ribs in and down, roll your inner arms out and squeeze your shoulder blades together. Keep your head and neck loose and free. Breathe in through your nose and out through your mouth saying, *"Haaaa."*

Be curious about any pain you feel. Consider your ancestors and what caused them pain as you feel the stretch. Hold as long as you can. Come out when you need to by walking your hands down your thighs to the floor and back under your shoulders to all fours.

On all fours, pick up your feet and gently tap your toes on the floor.

Strengthening – The Feet

Down Dog Taking a Walk –

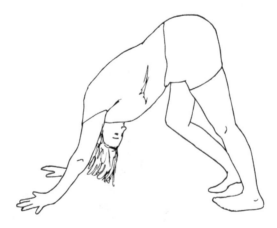

From all fours, with your hands under your shoulders and your knees under your hips, roll your inner arms out and squeeze your shoulder blades together. Tuck your toes under, lift your knees and come into a down dog by lifting your ribs in and down toward your pelvic bowl to engage your abdominals.

Bend one knee as you press through the opposite outer edge of the heel. Go for a slow walk. When ready, press both heels into the floor and breathe in through your nose and out through your mouth saying, *"Haaaa."* Honor the walk your ancestors took to bring you into this beautiful life you live.

Come out by walking your hands toward your feet. Hang and look at your feet while thanking your ancestors for the opportunity to experience this life.

Answer the Feet Inquiry Questions only after working on your feet.

Inquiry Questions: The Feet

These questions are designed to get you thinking beyond the physical manifestation of your low-back pain.

Your feet represent your ancestral energy. The right foot represents Dad's ancestors and the left foot represents Mom's ancestors.

You will be answering "what" questions. Not how, who, when, or where, because the mind answers those questions. The body answers the question "what." Please write down the first thing that comes into your mind as you read the question. Don't think about the questions or analyze your answers. Let the body answer, not your mind.

The Feet Questions

What is your greatest fear?

What is your relationship with food?

What do you do to nourish yourself?

The Feet Trauma Questions

What was your birth like? Did you experience any birth trauma?

What abandonment experiences have you had? Do you abandon yourself?

What is your experience of neglect? Do you neglect yourself?

Standing and Walking Questions
Look down at your feet as you stand. What do you notice?

What direction do your feet go when you stand?

Are they ducking out?
If yes, what are you controlling?

Are they pigeon-toeing in?
If yes, what boundaries do you need to set to feel safe in your world?

Are you placing weight on the balls of your feet?
If yes, what causes you to live more in the future than in the present moment?

Are your toes gripping the earth? If yes, what don't you trust?

Spend a Moment with Your Feet
What are they saying to you?

The Feet - Ancestral Questions
What were/are your dad's ancestors like? Describe them in as much detail as you can, focusing on both their strengths and weaknesses.

What were/are your mom's ancestors like? Describe them in as much detail as you can, focusing on both their strengths and weaknesses.

What diseases or disorders did or do your ancestors have?

What diseases or disorders that challenged your ancestors do you struggle with?

What was your ancestors' general emotional state?

What ancestral emotional states do you struggle with?

The Feet Pain Questions
What part or parts of your feet cause you pain?

What are you doing to alleviate your foot pain?

Look your answers over and consider the main things you learned about yourself from doing this questionnaire. What did you learn? Jot down your answers.

Now, we will move up to the next foundational point of the body, the legs.

The Legs Movement Practice
You'll need a softball-sized ball, block, Noodle Ball, strap, and your yoga mat.
A reminder:

- Do what you can. If something is too challenging, don't do it and make a note in the book, as it was designed as a workbook.
- Make a note of the exercises and practices that have the greatest impact on you.
- Remember the *Haaaa* Breath. Use it while you do each practice.

Ball Work – Legs

Ball in Your Inner Leg –

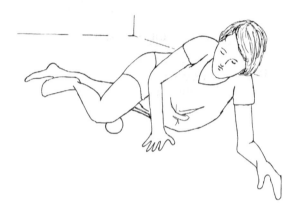

Place a softball-sized ball in your inner leg (groin area) in the gracilis muscle. Move your leg up toward your chest and down toward your bottom as you roll down your inner leg to your knee. If you don't feel much, place the ball up on a block. Switch sides and do the same thing on the other side.

This releases held anger that is stored in your inner leg. Your right inner leg holds anger toward the outer world which is taught to you by your dad. Your left inner leg holds anger toward yourself which is taught to you by your mom.

Noodle Ball Down Your Quads –

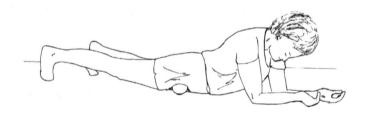

Place the noodle ball at the top of your quads (upper thigh). Roll down to your knee, rocking to the outer edge of your leg to release your IT Bands.

This movement releases the fight, flight, or freeze response held in your quads. The right side is responding to fear of things outside of you. The left side is responding to fear of your inner world.

The IT Band is located on the outer edge of your leg. This release will allow you to let go of your protective armor. On the right side, you are protecting yourself from "them." On the left side, you are protecting yourself from YOU!

Ball Down the Back of Your Legs –

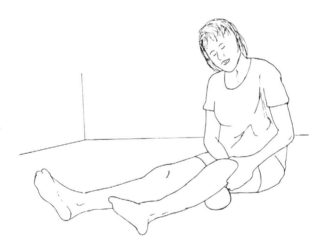

Sit with legs in front of you, then tuck a softball-sized ball under one leg, right at the top of the leg. Rock your legs side to side to move the ball to the outer leg and back to the inner leg. As you rock the leg side to side, slowly move the ball down your leg to the knee and the calf, ending at your ankle. As you roll, release whatever you are still holding onto from childhood. The right leg represents Dad's teaching on how to live in the outer world and the left leg represents Mom's teaching of how to be in your inner world.

The leg is a timeline — the top of the leg represents the age you were when you left home and went out on your own. As you roll the ball side to side, working your way down your leg, you go through the teenage years. The back of the knee represents pre-teen, the calf is early childhood, and the ankle is the point of conception.

All the pains and tensions you find with this ball work are from holding onto something from childhood that hurt you, didn't work for you or you didn't know how to process.

Breathe out the tension and pain with the *Haaaa* Breath and breathe in love!

Stretches – The Legs

Lying Leg Opener –

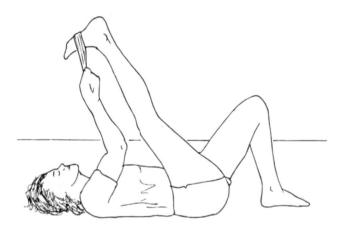

Lie on your back with your knees bent and your feet on the floor. Take your right knee to your chest and place a strap on the ball of your right foot. Exhale and extend through your heel, opening the back of your leg. Inhale, bend your knee and do this several times until you are ready to hold the extension.

As you hold, roll your inner leg in, press your heel to the sky, and take your toes down. With each exhalation bring your thigh closer to your belly until you reach the edge of the stretch (the end of your comfort zone; as far as you can go) in your hamstrings (the back of your leg). Hold and breathe.

When ready, place the strap in your right hand, keep your right leg straight and strong and lower your right foot toward the floor to the right. Don't allow your pelvis on the right side to lift off the ground. Feel the stretch in your gracilis muscle (the inner leg), hold the edge of this stretch, and breathe.

When ready, exhale your straight, strong leg back to center, switch hands and bring your left hand onto your strap. Exhale and bring your right foot to the left and your left knee to the right. Don't let your pelvis leave the floor on the right side. Feel the stretch in your IT band (the outer edge of your leg) and hold the edge of this stretch and breathe.

Come out, switch sides, and do the same thing on the other side.

This movement will open you to respect your parents and appreciate their teachings while releasing what doesn't work for you.

Release your Quads –

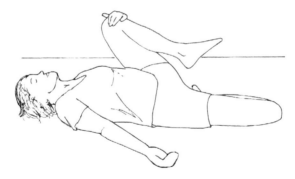

Lie on your back and hug both knees into your chest. Hold and breathe.

Drop your right foot to the floor and walk it to the left, even with your left mid-butt cheek. Drop your right knee to the floor and pull your left knee to your chest. Brush off your fear response to the outer world from your right thigh with your right hand. When ready, move your left leg around to go into different aspects of tension in your right quad muscles. Hold and breathe on these points of tension.

To come out, hug both knees into your chest. Hold and breathe. Release your held fear responses of fight, flight, or freeze.

Switch sides and do the same thing on the other side.

All Fours –

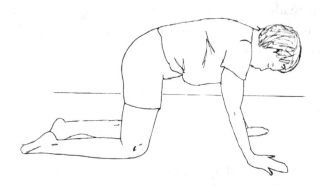

Come into a cat by bringing your knees under your hips and your hands under your shoulders on all fours. Bring your ribs up and in toward your pelvis, roll your inner arms out and squeeze your scapula together, while keeping a long lower back. From there, you can move your head and neck around and circle your hips in both directions.

Lunge to Runner's Stretch –

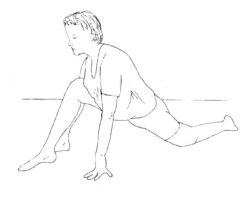

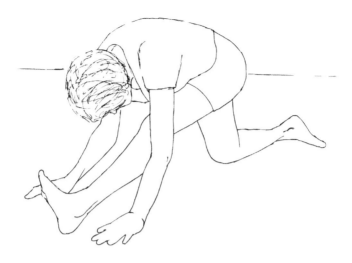

From all fours with your hands under your shoulders and your knees under your hips. Roll your inner arms out, lift your ribs up and in toward your spine and down toward your hip bones.

Hold your low-back in this position as you step your right leg forward. Walk your right leg as far forward as possible. If you need one, use a block to prop up your right hand. Exhale, drop your tail down and forward keeping your ribs in and down. Inhale, open your heart. Lift your head only as far as you can without creating wrinkles on the back of your neck.

Keep breathing in through your nose and out through your mouth. When ready, straighten your front leg. Keep your pelvis even, roll your inner leg in, push through your heel and bring your toes back to look at your body. Drop your belly toward your thigh and your chest toward your knees. Keep your head loose and free. Hold and breathe, and when ready come back to lunge. Do this at least two times.

When ready to come out, go back to all fours, switch sides, and do the same thing on the other side.

This pose will open the back of your legs and release your fear responses so you can respect your parents and bring in the energy of forgiveness.

Strengthening – The Legs

Downward Facing Dog –

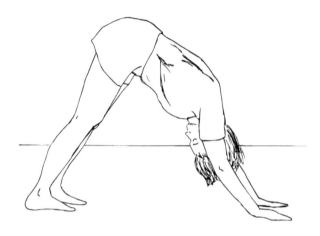

From all fours with your hands under your shoulders and your knees under your hips. Roll your inner arms out and squeeze your shoulder blades together. Take your toes under, lift your knees, and come into a down dog by lifting your ribs in and back toward your pelvic bowl.

Press both heels into the floor and breathe in through your nose and out through your mouth saying, *"Haaaa."* Hold and breathe.

Come out by walking your hands toward your feet. Hang and look at your feet and legs. Honor your ancestors and respect your parents.

Inquiry Questions: The Legs

These questions are designed to get you thinking beyond the physical manifestation of your low-back pain.

The legs represent the teachings of Mom and Dad. The right leg represents dad's teachings on how to be in the outer world. The left leg represents mom's teachings on how to be in your inner world of feelings and intuition.

Reminder: Please write out the first thing that comes into your mind; don't think about the questions too much.

The Legs Questions
What have you manifested for yourself?

What is your relationship with money?

What do you trust?

What do you mistrust?

What do you do when you need to set boundaries?

The Legs Trauma Questions
What forms of abuse have you experienced?

What accidents have you had?

What illnesses have you had, or do you currently have?

What surgeries have you had?

What traumas have you inherited?

What is your relationship with your body?

Standing and Walking
Look down at your legs as you stand before a mirror.

What do you notice?

What direction do your knees go when you stand?

Are they turned out?
If yes, what causes you to give up your inner truth?

What is your greatest strength?

Are they turning in?
If yes, What causes you to release your boundaries?

Are your legs sturdy and strong?

Are your legs weak?

Do you feel grounded?

Spend a Moment with Your Legs
What are they saying to you?

What would you describe your legs as energetically —

Deficient? Were you neglected or abandoned in childhood?

Excessive? Were you stressed out or smothered in childhood?

Or balanced somewhere in the middle, between deficient and excessive?

The Legs - Your Parents
What is/was your dad like? Describe him in as much detail as possible including his strengths and weaknesses.

What was/is your mom like? Describe her in as much detail as possible, including her strengths and weaknesses.

What diseases or disorders did or do your parents have?

What diseases or disorders that your parents had/have do you struggle with?

What was or is your parents' primary emotional state? Mom? Dad?

What is your primary emotional state?

Leg Pain
What parts of your legs cause you pain?

What are you doing to alleviate the pain and tension in your legs?

Look your answers over and consider the main things you learned about yourself from doing this questionnaire. What did you learn? Jot down your answers.

Anatomy of Your Gracilis Muscle and The Sciatic Nerve

The Anger Muscle — The Gracilis

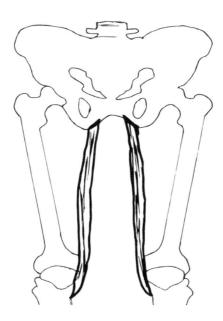

In the leg practices, you'll encounter the space in your body where you hold unprocessed anger, the **gracilis muscle**. The gracilis runs from your inner leg to your inner knee. It attaches at the front of the pelvis on the ischiopubic ramus and inserts into the tibia, the lower leg bone.

This muscle is meant to support your pelvis, but when weak, stuck, or tight, it causes the low-back to be hypermobile, causing the pelvis, sacrum, and lumbar vertebrae to go out of alignment.

This misalignment can cause your sacroiliac joint to dislocate and lumbar discs to bulge, herniate or dislocate, which can cause nerves to get pinched and muscles to tighten and spasm.

The gracilis also affects your feet. When this muscle is weak and tight, it can cause you to lose the inner arch of your foot and your feet to flatten, creating ankle, knee, hip, pelvis, and low-back challenges.

As you open and release the gracilis muscle, you will release held anger and allow the pelvic bowl, sacrum, and lumbar vertebrae to realign, easing out muscle tension and releasing pinched nerves.

And you'll get the arch back in your feet to further support your low-back.

The Sciatic Nerve

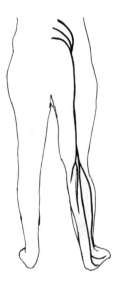

Many of you with low-back pain will experience sciatica. What is sciatica? Any type of pain and/or neurological symptom that originates from the sciatic nerve is referred to as sciatica. The symptoms of sciatica are typically felt along the path of the nerve and are caused by low-back challenges or butt-cheek clenching.

The sciatic nerve is the largest in the human body: the union of 5 nerve roots from the lower spine. It passes deep into the buttock and down the back of the thigh, all the way to the heel and sole of the foot. The sciatic nerve serves a vital role in connecting the spinal cord to the skin and muscles of the thigh, leg, and foot.

Your Pain-Free Low-Back Posture Daily Practice can release sciatica as it will take pressure off the sciatic nerve.

A Pain-Free Low-Back Story –

Lourdes was getting ready to move from California to Miami. She was worried that she wouldn't be able to pack up her house and physically make the transition because of the pain in her right butt cheek and leg caused by sciatica.

I assessed Lourdes' low-back and found that she had a combination of severe lordosis and tight glutes and piriformis (control) muscles. She began to do the work that I suggested and quickly got out of her low-back pain.

Lourdes was still experiencing some sciatica, but as she kept doing her daily practice it slowly released as well. Here's what Lourdes said, *Oh my gosh, I was in so much pain I really didn't think I could handle our big move to Miami – but within a month I was out of low-back pain. Slowly my sciatica began to release until I couldn't believe it but I was out of pain, packing boxes, and getting ready to move!*

Chapter 11 – Let Go of Your Hips, Glutes, Piriformis, and Control to Create Stability

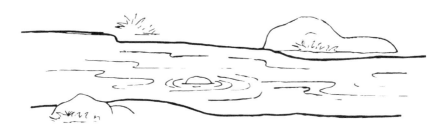

Create, create it's what you are here to do!
Jen Healey

You continue to build your Pain-Free Low-Back Posture Daily Practice as you let go of the grip of control held in your butt cheeks, piriformis, and hip flexors. Let go of control so your creativity flows.

Hips, Glutes, and Piriformis Movement Practice

You'll need your yoga mat, softball-sized ball, and wall space.

A reminder:

- Do what you can. If something is too challenging, don't do it and make a note in the book, as it was designed as a workbook.
- Make a note of the exercises and practices that have the greatest impact on you.
- Remember the *Haaaa* Breath. Use it while you do each practice.

Ball work - Hips, Glutes, and Piriformis

Softball-sized Ball in Your Butt Cheeks –

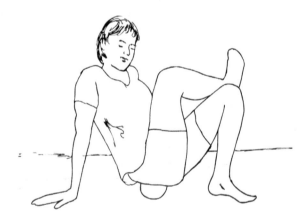

Lie down or sit up with the ball under your right butt cheek, with your right ankle on your left knee. Roll around finding knots of tension. Stay on the knots and move back and forth over them, breathing out the desire to control others.

Switch sides after two minutes and place the ball in your left butt cheek, with your left ankle on your right knee. Roll around finding knots of tension. Stay on the knots and move back and forth over them breathing out control of yourself.

Stretches - Hips, Glutes, and Piriformis

Butt Cheek Stretch —

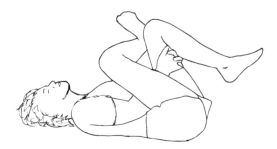

Lie on your back and place your right ankle on your left knee. Place your hands on the back of your left thigh and draw your left knee toward your chest. Find your edge (the end of your comfort zone; as far as you can go), then hold and breathe. Let go of control of your outer world and breathe in acceptance of whatever comes your way.

When ready, switch sides and place the left ankle on the right knee. On this side, breathe out letting go of control of yourself and breathe in acceptance.

Fire Log –

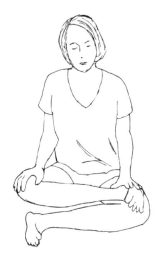

From sitting cross-legged, take your right ankle in line with your right knee. Pick up your left leg, lift the calf up toward your heart and rock your leg left to right. When ready, set your left ankle on your right knee and press your left knee toward your right ankle with your left hand positioned slightly above your left knee. You may need to place your bottom on a pillow or block or leave your hand/arm behind you. If you can, keep pressing your left knee down, come forward and rest your chest toward your calves. Hold and Breathe. Let go of control. When ready, come out, switch sides, and do the same thing on the other side. If this is too hard for you, do it sitting in a chair!!

Pigeon Pose –

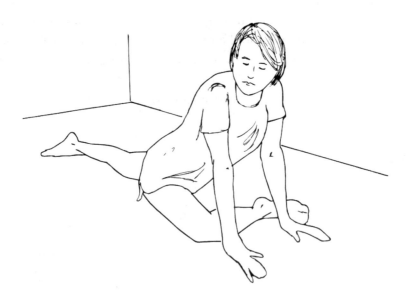

From all fours, take your right ankle to the outer edge of your left knee. Walk your left leg back until your bottom is as close to the floor as possible. Place a pillow under your bottom if your bottom is off the floor or your knee hurts. Drop to your elbows. Hang your head and breathe, release control. Switch sides and do the same thing on the other side.

Strengthening - Hips, Glutes, and Piriformis

Standing Hip and Butt Cheek Release –

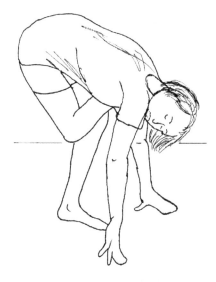

Start with your feet inner hip-width apart. Push into the outer edges of your heels. Take your tail down, ribs in and down, and roll your inner arms out. Hold and breathe.

Come to stand on your left foot. Use a wall for balance if needed. When ready, bend your standing knee and place your right ankle on your left knee. Come forward and if you can, take your hands to the floor or to a block or chair if needed. Continue bending your standing leg until you feel a good stretch in your right butt cheek. Hold and breathe, letting go of the desire to control.

When ready to come out, come back up to standing, switch sides, and do the same thing on the other side.

This practice will release your piriformis muscle (the control muscle of the body), allowing you to accept everything just as it is. "*Haaaa!*"

What are Your Unique Gifts and Talents?

We are all given inborn gifts and talents. It is important to know yours so that you can use them to live a productive, rich life. When you squeeze your butt cheeks, you stop the flow of your natural gifts and talents to the point that you may not even be aware of what they are.

Let's dive into understanding what your gifts and talents truly are, so that you can own them and use them to live your life to the fullest.

Answer the following questions to understand and own your gifts and talents.

What did you love to do as a child?

How would you pass your summer days?

What types of activities did you find exciting?

What are you passionate about now?

What motivates you?

What do you do that you get totally lost in?

What kind of "geek" are you?

What are the main topics of the books on your bookshelf?

What do you enjoy reading? (*This is how I figured out that I wanted to become a yoga therapist. All of the books that I was reading were on the topic of yoga or therapy*).

What puzzles you that you want to figure out?
Is it people, complicated life situations, or building a better widget?

Perhaps the Universe, God, or spiritual matters?

Maybe the environment, climate change, or nature in general?

Or how to ski, skate, write, paint, or a thousand other things?

Ask your family, friends, and co-workers. Think of the five people you spend the most time with and ask them to share with you what they think your gifts, talents, qualities, and strengths are.

You could get the person that you are closest with to answer this question: What I like and admire about (YOU!!) is _____.

Remember - This list is NOT about a pursuit you've perfected. It's something you love to do, create, and get lost in. You love to talk endlessly about it, time slips away and you bliss out when you do it.

It could be anything that you love to do!! Watching your kids or grandkids play, baking cookies, figuring out how to make a fancy bun in your hair, figure drawing, teaching swing dancing, or singing show tunes. It could also be climbing rocks, chasing tornados, talking about music, playing the ukulele, or riding your bike with no hands. I could go on and on.

It's just the thing that you love to do and are most passionate about!! **What is that? Write it down, shout it out, and OWN it!!** It's yours — your thing. Love it!!

A NOTE: No one else is going to embrace you for that thing that you love to do until you own your gifts and rock your talents!

Why You Should Use Your Talents or Gifts

*"Hide not your talents, they for use were made, What's
a sundial in the shade?"* Benjamin Franklin

Our gifts or talents are also considered our strengths. Gallup researched people who use their strengths every day and how it affects their performance and overall quality of life. They found that people who use their gifts and talents (something that comes naturally and can be enhanced through practice) every day are six times more likely to be engaged in life.

The research concluded that those who use their strengths and talents experience:

a. Improved health and wellness
b. Less worry, stress, anger, sadness, or physical pain
c. A boost to their positive emotions
d. More energy to face the day
e. Higher engagement level

They also found out that supporting people's gifts and talents, which are their strengths, is a far more effective approach to improving performance than trying to "fix" weaknesses.

Gallup's data shows that simply identifying their strengths makes people 7.8% more productive.

This means YOU can benefit from using your gifts and talents (strengths) every day.

Are you using your gifts and talents every day?

How can you start to use them daily?

What have you created in your lifetime?

We've all created many things in our lifetimes. Whether you created consciously using your gifts and talents, or you unconsciously created based on circumstances and opportunity, it is important to honor your creations.

Take about five minutes to think of the things that you've created in your life and list them below:

Go back into your list and circle everything that you have created by consciously using your gifts, talents, and strengths.

Put stars by the things that you are most proud of.

Allow yourself to sit with each starred creation and feel the joy.

What do you want to create?

No matter how old you are, you are still here to create.

One of my students, Terry Cohen, didn't begin to create her life's dream until she was in her seventies. Terry loves hunting for treasures. It is her talent and she is very gifted at finding unique, special, and rare items.

At seventy, Terry created a store called Curiosities to display and sell her special finds. It has been open for thirteen years now and is very successful. Her store is THE place to go to find that unique piece that you can't find anywhere else. Terry's been interviewed in magazines and newspapers for creating a shop like no other.

Just think if Terry had stopped herself from creating her life's dream because she was "too old." The world would have missed out on a truly unique shopping experience.

Make sure you don't block yourself from creating as long as you are alive.

List the thing or things you would like to create in your life:

Are you in the process of creating it or them?

What stops you from making your dreams come true?

List one thing you can do TODAY to make your dream creations a reality.

Commit to doing just one thing a day to create your dreams. Are you in?

Anatomy of the Piriformis

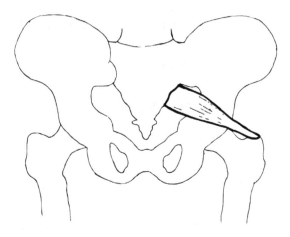

The Control Muscle — The Piriformis

To get your gifts and talents flowing and to make your dreams come true, you've got to release your piriformis muscle and address your control issues.

The piriformis muscle runs beneath your gluteus maximus (large butt muscle). When you want something to be different than it is (my definition of control), the piriformis grabs and shoves your sacrum into your lower back.

Your sacrum is meant to release down so that the lumbar vertebrae have space between them. You have to release your piriformis to let go of the sacrum and allow it to drop away from the lumbar vertebrae. Once you do this, your low-back can decompress and be free.

Your sciatic nerve runs diagonally to your piriformis, or in some people right through it, so piriformis tension can tangle or squeeze on the sciatic nerve, causing sciatica.

Inquiry Questions: The Hips, Glutes, and Piriformis

These questions are designed to get you thinking beyond the physical manifestation of your low-back pain.

Your hips and butt cheeks represent control. Again, my definition of control is wanting something or somebody to be different from the way it is. The brain can't decipher between wishing something was different and consciously attempting to make something different than it is.

Reminder: You will be answering "what" questions. Write down the first thing that comes to mind as you read the question. Don't think about the questions. Let the body answer, not the mind.

Dive deep with curiosity into uncovering what causes you to grip your butt cheeks and tighten your hips.

The Hips, Glutes, and Piriformis Questions

What or who are you trying to control?

What is the level of tension that you hold in your butt cheeks?

What is your sex life like? Is it pleasurable?

What do you struggle with sexually?

What are the reasons that you make love?

What best describes you? Impulsive or compulsive?

What is the state of your most intimate relationship? Do you feel nurtured, respected, and heard?

What are you willing to risk for your dream(s) to come true? What would you risk for love? What would you risk to be your best self?

What are you willing to let go of so that your dreams can manifest?

What or who do you trust to support you? What or who shares your dreams?

What or who do you turn to when the going gets tough?

What bothers you about someone else? What shadow aspect of yourself is that person showing you?

What is your experience with sexual abuse?

What is your experience with rape?

What is your experience with abortion?

Spend a Moment with Your Hips, Glutes, and Piriformis
Are your butt cheeks squeezed together? Gently tap them to see if they release. Can they let go?

Hips, Glutes, and Piriformis Trauma Questions
What pain do you have in your hips?

What do you want to control (wish was different than it is) so much that you can't let it go?

Look your answers over and consider the main things that you learned about yourself from doing this questionnaire. What did you learn? Jot down your answers.

Now, we will move on to making your dreams come true.

The Simple Steps to Make Your Dreams Come True

Own Your Gifts and Talents
My gifts and talents are:_____
_____.

Start referring to yourself as your gift — for example, say — I am a teacher, an artist, an actress, an organizer, a fund-raiser, a connector, a dancer, a mother, a lover…whatever your gift is!

I am a _____
_____.

Build a Plan

Harvey MacKay put it best when he said, *"A dream is just a dream, a goal is a dream with a plan and a deadline."*

You've got to build a plan to get you from where you are to where you want to go. It will keep you on track and minimize the detours that slow or delay your progress toward your goal.

So, if your dream is to write your first book, your plan could be to get up an hour earlier to write one thousand words before going about your day. That way, when you set your alarm each night, you know what time to set it for. When you wake up, you'll know that it's time to do your daily practice, open up the laptop, and get typing.

One of the great things about a plan is that it helps you to track your progress along the way.

What is the one thing that you are going to do every day to make your dreams come true? _____
_____.

Set a Deadline

Deadlines work magic. When set, they stop procrastination in their tracks and whip you into gear so that you start getting things done.

Even though you have a plan, you may spend lots and lots of time thinking that you need to learn more, or worried that your plan isn't just right, or if you need to go check Facebook again (you don't). And then you'll wake up, look at the calendar, months will have passed, and you'll have barely moved an inch toward your goal.

But a deadline changes all of that. Because you know you can't miss it, you do what you need to do to get things done.

So give yourself a due date. And then tell someone who will hold you accountable. Be sure to permit them to kick your butt.

What is your deadline? _____

_____.

Who's going to keep you accountable? _____.

By (date) _____, *I will* _____

_____ *(have a book draft, develop healthy eating habits, etc.)*

Do the Work

There's no way around this: You've got to work on your plan.

Push yourself to do it when you feel like working. More importantly, push yourself to do it when you don't feel like working.

Consistency yields results, and then you can move on to the next step.

Celebrate!

Dreams don't usually come true in one day. Reaching goals takes time. Sometimes you'll need a bit of encouragement along the way to keep you going. So, whenever you hit certain milestones, stop what you're doing, take a pause, and give yourself a high-five for all the progress you've made.

You deserve it, and although you may not be exactly where you want to go, you are further than when you started. That's worth celebrating. It's also fuel to persevere.

It's Time to Make Your Dreams a Reality

Your dreams don't have to stay just dreams — they can become your reality. But the majority of the time, dreams come true only as a result of us doing what's necessary to make them happen.

By owning your gifts, building a plan, setting a deadline, and doing the work, you'll look back a year from now (maybe sooner) at all that you have accomplished and smile.

Because you'll know that dreams do come true.

Because yours finally did.

Chapter 12 - Free Fear From Your Quads and Iliopsoas to Connect to The Emotional Guidance System

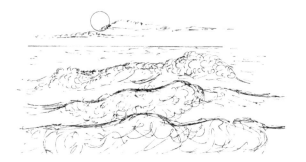

This being human is a guest house.
Every morning a new arrival.
A joy, a depression, a meanness,
some momentary awareness comes
as an unexpected visitor.
Welcome and entertain them all!
Rumi

Continue building your Pain-Free Low-Back Posture Daily Practice by opening your iliopsoas and quad muscles to release held fear.

Letting go of fear allows your emotions to move freely up to joy or down to depression.

Let's get your inner guidance system up and running again.

Emotional Guidance System (EGS) Introduction and Mirroring Lesson

I love, love, LOVE sharing the Emotional Guidance System (EGS) work with others!

Most of you weren't taught how to use your feelings and intuition to guide you through your life. You are not alone. The majority of us are emotionally stunted because we came out of a patriarchal time where thinking was honored more than feeling.

When you learn what your emotions are and how to use them, life gets a whole lot simpler. Your feelings and intuition ease your lower back pain, hip pain, and pelvic pain. Why?? Because the pelvis and lower back are, energetically speaking, the containers of your emotions. When you are blocking feelings, you are setting up energy blocks in your pelvic bowl.

Your Emotional Guidance System (EGS)

The sole purpose of your emotions and intuition is to guide you through your life. When you feel something, it's either a positive emotion going up toward joy or a negative emotion going down toward depression.

Road map

Your feelings are like a road map. To travel by car from NYC to LA you have to make many stops. From New York City to Toledo, OH, to Chicago, IL, to Des Moines, IA, to Omaha, NE, to Denver, CO, to Las Vegas, NV, then finally arriving in Los Angeles.

Your feelings are the same way. Let's say you are depressed. You will have to pass through many feelings: from depression/anxiety to anger, to frustration, to feeling overwhelm, to pessimism, to pessimistic optimism, to optimism, to hope, to faith, to trust, to happiness, before finally – hopefully –, you arrive at joy.

When you are taught to block emotions, it's like running into a "Road Closed" sign on the freeway. You have to turn around and emotionally go back down the emotional scale. That's why many of you feel the same feelings over and over again. You may be going toward joy, but you aren't supposed to feel anger, so you go right back to depression.

When something happens to trigger frustration, to move to joy, you have to go through many emotions on the "map" from frustration to joy. You have to feel every one of those emotions that you were taught not to feel.

So, how do we do that?

Mirroring

Your mother was meant to teach you how to use your inner guidance system through mirroring. For example, if you were yelling because someone broke your toy, your mother might have gotten down to your level and mimicked you shouting and clenching your fists. She might have said something like, "Shouting, you are shouting because you are angry. I hear you and see your clenched fists. You must be angry that your toy broke. Let's see if we can fix it." From that mirroring, you then came to understand that when you shout and clench your fists, that means you are angry.

You lose anger as a valid emotion and begin to repress it when your mother says, "Don't shout, settle down, your toy just broke. Get over it."

To reinstate your Emotional Guidance System (EGS) you need to mirror your emotions back to yourself. You are going to do this by making an Emotional Guidance System (EGS). You will create a set of emotional images and use them during an emotional movement meditation.

Make your EGS

You're going to get creative. Your pelvis is your creative center, so you are going to connect with your creative gifts and talents to create your emotional guidance system.

Get out your crayons and paints. Gather a stack of magazines to find images or find and print out photos on the internet. You could get out your camera and go into nature to find images as well. You'll also need thick art paper, cardboard or index cards, and glue.

You are going to find or make an external image that represents each emotion. They will include:

Depression/Anxiety/Fear - Anger - Frustration - Overwhelm - Pessimism - Pessimistic Optimism - Optimism - Hope - Faith - Trust - Happiness - Joy

I realize that every single emotion is not included on this list; that's to keep this exercise as simple as possible.

Pick out the colors, the words, and the images that match each emotion and paste or sketch them on your separate drawings, so that each drawing you've created represents the feeling inside. Your drawing of anger needs only to represent anger to you. ONLY you!! Don't get other opinions on your EGS!

Here are a few quick sketches and definitions of my feelings for "inspiration."

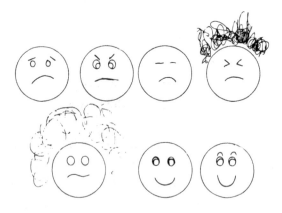

Depression, Anxiety, and Fear

Depression is a feeling of sadness or loss of interest in pleasurable activities. It feels inescapable and is the heaviest/darkest human feeling you can have.

Anxiety is excessive nervousness, apprehension, and worry.

Fear is signaled by a racing heart, sweaty palms, and feelings of panic. These feelings alert you to danger. You don't want to hang on to fear once you're safely out of the scary situation. Acute fear is okay, but chronic fear is not.

These are all heavy human emotions. (As a reminder, as you go up the emotional scale you transition from heavy human emotions to lighter, spiritual emotions).

Anger

Anger is an emotion characterized by antagonism toward someone or something that you feel has deliberately done you wrong.

Anger can be a good thing. It can give you a way to express negative feelings or motivate you to find solutions to problems. It can move you out of depression. It is a heavy human emotion.

I get angry when my needs aren't met. The anger fuels my power to do something about my situation so that I can meet my needs. Anger is a human emotion.

Frustration

Frustration is the feeling of being upset or annoyed, especially because of an inability to change or achieve something. It is a heavy human emotion.

I relate frustration to that low-level *grrrrrr* that I feel when something's amiss in my life and I feel powerless to change it. Frustration is a human emotion.

Overwhelm and Stress

Overwhelm and stress feel like you are going to be buried or drowned beneath something heavy.

I feel overwhelmed and stressed when I'm too busy working or have too many projects on my list of things to do. It is a human emotion.

Pessimism

Pessimism is a tendency to see the worst aspect of things or believe that the worst will happen; a lack of hope or confidence in the future.

This negativity invades me when things take too long to change. It is a human emotion.

Pessimistic Optimism

Pessimistic optimism is feeling like you need to plan ahead because you know to expect the unexpected. It could go all wrong, so you're always prepared for the worst, but it could go all right, too. It is a human/spiritual emotion.

I often feel this when I'm about to do something that I've never done before.

Optimism

Optimism is hopefulness and confidence about the future or the successful outcome of something. It is a spiritual emotion.

I feel optimistic when I've done something that I've never done before and I've come through it successfully.

Hope

Hope is a feeling of expectation and desire for a certain thing to happen. It is a spiritual emotion.

I feel hopeful when I sense progress in difficult situations.

Faith

Faith is complete confidence in someone or something. It is a spiritual emotion.

I have faith when people's words and actions line up.

Trust

Trust is a firm belief in the reliability, truth, ability, or strength of someone or something. It is a spiritual emotion.

I trust people and situations that remain constantly steady in my life.

Happiness

Happiness is that feeling that comes over you when you know life is good and you can't help but smile. It is a spiritual emotion.

I feel happy when I'm walking on the beach, going hiking in beauty, snorkeling with the fish, and helping people out of low-back pain. I feel satisfied and content.

Joy

Joy is the feeling of great delight. It is a spiritual emotion.

I've experienced joy when in nature. It's a feeling of complete happiness, and ease with vulnerability.

Begin to create your Emotional Guidance System! You'll learn so much about yourself through the process. And in between working on your EGS, move fear out of your body!

The Iliopsoas and Quads Movement Practice

You'll need your yoga mat, softball-sized ball, and wall space.

A reminder:

- Do what you can. If something is too challenging, don't do it and make a note in the book, as it was designed as a workbook.
- Make a note of the exercises and practices that have the greatest impact on you.
- Remember the *Haaaa* Breath. Use it while you do each practice.

Ball Work - The Iliopsoas and Quads

Ball in Your Iliopsoas and Quads –

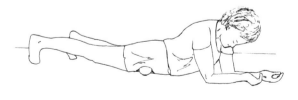

Lie on your belly. (This may hurt your low back initially. Keep doing it if the pain isn't too severe). Place a softball-sized ball into the inside of your right hip bone. Roll toward your pubic bone and back toward your hip bone. Your iliopsoas will be the place that feels a bit painful. I describe the iliopsoas pain as feeling like a screechy violin. When you feel that, you know that you are in the right place.

Roll slowly down and into your inguinal crease, the top of your leg, about halfway to your inner groin. The right iliopsoas represents fear of the outer world, others, and situations outside of yourself. Breathe out the fear of others and breathe in gratitude.

Keep rolling the ball down to your quads, across to the outer leg, back to the inner leg, and down to above your knee. The quads hold your fear response: flight, fight or freeze. Breathe out your held fear responses and breathe in freedom.

When ready, it's time to do the left side the same way that you did your right side, adding breathing out the fear of yourself and breathing in gratitude for your authentic self.

Stretching - The Iliopsoas and Quads

Hug Your Knees –

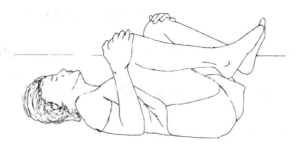

Lie on your back and bring your knees to your chest. Gently hug your knees and breathe deeply in and out of your belly. Feel your knees dropping into your body as you exhale and moving away from your body as you inhale. Rest here feeling the gentle rocking motion.

When ready, make circles slowly going in both directions. You can also rock gently from side to side. Breathe as you rock and/or circle. **This pose can bring you a tremendous amount of relief from low-back pain.**

Iliopsoas Quad Opener –

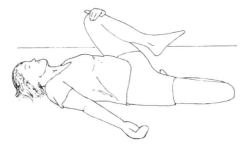

From lying down, bring your knees to your chest. On an exhalation, bring your left foot to the floor, keeping your right knee in toward your chest. Walk your left foot to the right. Drop your left knee to the floor as you pull your left heel into the center of your right butt cheek with you right hand. Hold and breathe letting go of fear.

Switch sides and do the same thing on the other side.

All Fours –

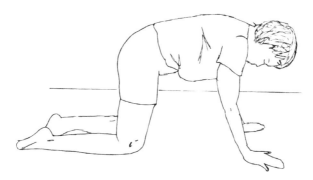

Come into a cat by bringing your knees under your hips and your hands under your shoulders on all fours. Bring your ribs up and in toward your pelvis, roll your inner arms out and squeeze your scapula together, keeping a long lower back. From there, you can move your head and neck around and circle your hips in both directions.

Lunge –

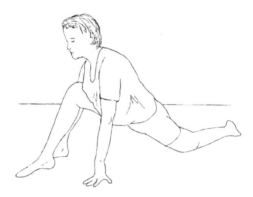

From all fours, step the right leg forward into a lunge. Walk the right foot as far forward as possible. Press your back foot into the earth and drop your pelvis down and forward. Roll the inner arms out. On each exhale drop your tail and on each inhale open your heart. Use a block if it's difficult to get your hands to the floor. On an exhale, pull your right knee into your chest. Turn your chest to your right knee, hold and breathe, dropping your tail down on each exhalation, no wrinkles on the back of the neck. Hold and breathe.

Switch sides and do the same thing on the other side.

Lunge With The Leg Up The Wall –

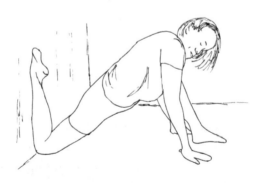

Come to a wall with a folded blanket set right up to the wall. Get on all fours facing away from the wall. Exhale and bring your left knee up the wall. Step your right foot forward and walk your foot as far forward as it will go. If your right foot can't step forward, just slide your right knee as far forward as you can. If you need to, use a block for your right hand. Exhale, drop your pelvis down and forward, no wrinkles on the back of your neck. Hold and breathe. When you're ready, come out by backing up your bottom and stepping your left knee forward. Rest, switch sides, and do the same thing on the other side.

Strengthening - The Iliopsoas and Quads

Down Dog –

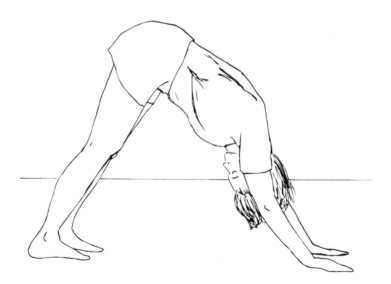

Go back to all fours with hands under shoulders, knees under hips, and ribs up and in. Roll your inner arms out as you squeeze your shoulder blades together. Exhale, lift your knees, and come up to Down Dog, pressing your heels to (or toward) the floor. Hold and breathe for about two minutes.

Down Dog With The Leg Back –

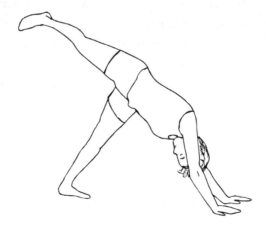

From Down Dog, lift your right leg straight up and back behind you, pressing through your right heel. Lift your right hip to the sky, then drop your straight strong right leg back behind you. Hold and breathe. When ready, switch sides and do the same thing on the other side. Let go of fear.

Forward Fold –

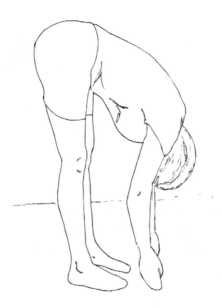

From standing, on an exhalation drop forward into a standing forward bend. Allow your upper body to be loose and free, your legs to flow down, your knees to be slightly bent and your feet to connect deeply to the earth. Push into the outer edge of your heels and spread your toes wide apart. Breathe and hold. Press into the outer edges of your heels to slowly come up. As you stand, bring your tail down, press your ribs in and down toward the pelvic bowl, and roll your inner arms out as you squeeze your shoulder blades together. Your head and neck are loose and free.

Standing Posture –

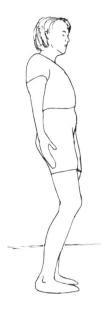

Stand with your feet inner hip-width apart, lined up from the inside of your hip bones. Press into the outer edge of your heels, lift and spread your toes, then set them down gently on the earth without gripping. Softly bend your knees as you feel your legs ground.

Allow your sacrum and tail to drop down and your ribs to snap in and down toward your pelvis. Roll your inner arms out and squeeze your scapula together, forming back cleavage. Breathe in and out of your open heart.

Standing Iliopsoas and Quad Release –

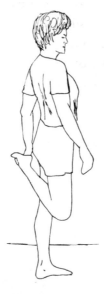

From standing, bring your weight onto your left foot, exhale, and draw your right knee to your chest. Pause and feel the length of your lower back. Take your right hand down your shin as you drop your knee toward the floor. Attempt to bring your knees even with one another while keeping a long lower back. Switch your grip to your left hand and bring your right heel toward your left buttocks. Breathe and flow on the waves of the breath as you hold. Exhale and come back to standing.

Switch sides and do the same thing on the other side.

Are You Stuck in Fight, Flight, or Freeze?

Your nervous system is an amazing communication network. It's time to understand how this powerful system works and what it takes to make it healthy.

By understanding how these survival instincts work, and noticing when they are "on" when they shouldn't be, you gain access to your very own personal medicine cabinet. I want to start by asking you a few questions:

Question #1 - When you encounter a mild, moderate, and/or severely stressful situation or harmful or traumatic event, what is your default pattern?

A) Do you tend to fight?

Do you:

- Get defensive and try to prove your case? (Even if you know you're wrong — you hold your ground anyway and would NEVER admit fault.)
- Raise your voice and display raging bull-like tendencies?
- Become a bit of a bully and even become scary to the people you love?

B) Do you tend to flee?

Do you:

- Ignore the situation and pretend it didn't happen?
- Leave the room or conversation and do your best to avoid any and all confrontations?
- Get busy and preoccupied with something completely unrelated to the situation at hand - you start cleaning, or go for a walk, etc … in the hope that it will just go away on its own?

C) Do you tend to freeze?

Do you:

- Go completely blank and find it hard to express ANYTHING, let alone engage in an argument or even respond?
- Hope that if you get really quiet, stay still, and don't make a peep, the aggressor or issue will just go away on its own?

- Completely forget a stressful or traumatic situation that happened to you? When someone asks you about it, you say, "What are you talking about?" (And sometimes you don't even recall the incident.)

D) All of the above:

Do you:

- Want to fight in some situations?
- Find yourself wanting to flee from others?
- Go completely blank and shut down?

Write in your response here:

Did you find that you had one distinct response (fight, flight, freeze); two, or did you find yourself experiencing all three?

Fact: These three responses - fight, flight, and freeze - are necessary. They are your SURVIVAL INSTINCTS kicking in. And you need them to alert you to danger. They keep you out of harm's way. You couldn't survive without them.

It's YOUR Nervous System, Your autonomic (automatic) nervous system, that governs these responses.

Your Survival Instincts in Action
Here are some basic real-life examples of these automatic stress responses in action.

A - Let's say that you're cutting carrots with bare feet and all of a sudden the knife slips out of your hands. The sharp blade is headed straight for your bare feet. But, in an INSTANT, and without conscious thought, you pull your foot out of the way and you miss the falling knife. This is a FLEE response.

This is your autonomic nervous system automatically working FOR YOU. It's keeping your body – in this case, your toes, and foot – safe.

B - Maybe you're out for a walk and some creepy person starts to harass you. You raise your voice a bit, square your shoulders to show your strength, and firmly tell this creep to leave.

That's your FIGHT response working for YOU.

C - Perhaps you are driving down the highway and you come across a bad accident. People are hurt as you see blood and bodies. You find it tough to look, but instead of averting your eyes, you stare directly at the grisly scene. Your body goes numb and you don't feel anything.

This is your FREEZE response working FOR YOU. It's not allowing you to feel the horror that you are witnessing.

I could give you many more examples, but I'm sure you get the idea. All you need to understand is that you've got these three automatic body responses: Fight, Flight, or, Freeze. They are a built-in system in your body, part of what is called the Autonomic Nervous System.

Question #2 - Can you think of a time when your survival instincts helped you out:

A. By getting you safely out of harm's way?

B. By giving you the courage to set a big boundary and show some healthy fight energy?

C. By fleeing to get away from a stressful or threatening situation?

D. By going into a freeze or shutdown after an accident?

Write in your response here:

These survival energies are fast-acting. All three responses (fight, flee, and freeze) ARE necessary and we need them to survive. However, once the trauma has passed they are meant to shut off, NOT be on 24/7.

These reactions are meant to stop once the stressor or threat or harmful event is over so that we can go back to normal easy functioning. Our body and its systems aren't built to stay in constant fight, flight, or freeze mode.

When we stay revved up in the fight, flight, or freeze survival mode, our stress hormones, adrenaline, and cortisol get overused and can become depleted.

Our current society doesn't support a low-stress lifestyle. Many of us are constantly ON and always on the GO. We are in trauma from Covid, war, political unrest, abuse, bullying, and accidents, and our fight, flight and freeze nervous system is chronically turned on.

If you grew up in a home that never felt safe, supportive, and secure, that was the perfect set-up for learning to keep your fight, flight, and freeze nervous system on high alert at all times. It is also the perfect set-up for many physical problems, including low-back pain.

Ask yourself:

1. How often do you feel stress and react using one of these three distinct survival instincts that I've been teaching you about?

   a. Once a day
   b. A few times (1 to 5) a day
   c. Many times (5 or more) a day
   d. All the time

Do you ever stop to notice them so that you can properly release the stress?

When we don't come down and out of our stress responses, we often end up with stress-related ailments.

Like low-back pain!

Our nervous system runs the show, and it doesn't always know how to come down and out of the fight, flight, and freeze modes. This constant state of "on guard," "under threat" and "survival" creates

TONS of INTERNAL STRESS, and it wreaks havoc on your body and low-back.

How do we stop this cycle?
The first step is awareness, which you've gained through the information and questions above.

The next step is connecting your mind and body with ball work and movements in the place where you hold your fight, flight, or flee responses – your quads.

As you work on your quads with awareness, your nervous system will shed fear responses. You'll release tightness and tension, allowing your low-back to decompress and your whole body to relax.

As you work on your quads, release the fear by breathing in through your nose and out through your mouth, saying, *"Haaaa"*. This sound will soothe and calm you.

Anatomy of Your Iliopsoas and Quads

The iliopsoas are made up of two muscles. It is the bottom part of the psoas muscle and blends in with the iliacus muscle as the psoas flows into the pelvic bowl.

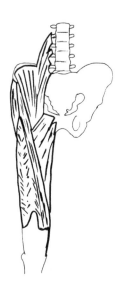

The psoas and the iliopsoas are the fear muscles of the body. All mammals have them. The psoas pulls the shoulders down and forward, and the iliopsoas draws the knees up and in to curl you into a ball to protect your soft underbelly from whatever is threatening you.

They are governed by the reptilian part of the brain, the brain stem, making it an instinctually reactive muscle.

The quads are the fear reactor muscles. When we are afraid, our bodies react with the flight, fight, or freeze response. As we get stuck in fear, our iliopsoas and quads get locked into these fear reactions. When the iliopsoas and quads get stuck in fear, they push the sacrum up into the low-back, compressing the low-back vertebrae. This compression can cause low-back pain resulting from discs, bulging discs, or degenerative disc disease.

To release low-back pain, we must undo the chronic contraction of the iliopsoas and quads so that the sacrum can fall away from the low-back.

EGS Meditation –

Once you have created your Emotional Guidance System (EGS), it is time for you to use it to move your emotions. Grab a timer and the images of your emotions. Sit in an open space where you can lay out the images of your emotions in front of you.

Place the images in front of you, starting with Depression, Anxiety, and Fear on the left-hand side, followed by Anger, Frustration, Overwhelm (Stress), Pessimism, Pessimistic/Optimism, Optimism, Hope, Faith, Trust, Happiness, and Joy in that ascending order, with the happy ones to the right.

Sit back, relax, and take three slow deep breaths.

Ask yourself, "What am I feeling right now?"

Look at the images of your emotions and choose the one that resonates the most with you. Pull the image of that emotion out (let's say it's anger) and place the image right in front of you.

Set your timer for ninety seconds and look at the image of that emotion (anger) as you connect with the feeling (anger) inside of you. If your mind wanders, go back to gazing at the image and feel that energy in your body (anger).

When the ninety seconds is up, move one emotion up from the emotion (anger) you were feeling. If you were feeling anger, move up to frustration.

Set your timer for ninety seconds and concentrate on the image of that emotion (frustration) as you connect with the feeling of that emotion (frustration) inside of you. If your mind wanders, go back to gazing at the image of the emotion and feeling that feeling (frustration).

Move just one emotion up. When you get good at shifting one emotion, you can easily shift all the way up the emotional scale.

Always move your emotions up toward joy!

Practice this meditation every day for a month or more until you get really good at moving up the emotional scale toward joy. As you practice moving one emotion up from wherever you find yourself at the moment, you become free to move up the emotional scale to joy.

You will no longer be stuck in emotions. Depression will lift, anxiety and fear will ebb away, stress will release, and you will let go of control. You will know how to regulate your emotions and move up the scale toward joy no matter what is going on around you or inside of you.

A Pain-Free Low-Back Story –

I looked at Trisha and noticed that she was living with tight ilio-psoas (fear) muscles on both sides. I also saw that on the right side of her low-back, her quadratus lumborum (stress) muscle was much tighter than on the left. Trisha had flat feet, indicating her gracilis (anger) muscle was not functioning.

I knew that Trisha needed to do the myofascial release ball work, stretching, and strengthening daily practice, but it was just as important that she reinstate her Emotional Guidance System.

This is what Trisha says: *"I'm a Brit and we are taught not to feel feelings. Then this lady Michelle comes along and tells me that my low-back pain is caused by holding onto feelings... well, I thought she was crazy. Listen to this crazy lady. She knows what she is talking about. In my opinion, The Emotional Guidance System work is the most important work you will do to release your low-back pain."*

Inquiry Questions: The Iliopsoas, Quads, and Low-Back

These questions are designed to get you thinking beyond the physical manifestation of your low-back pain.

The iliopsoas is the fear muscle, the quads the fear response muscle, and the low-back is the stress alarm bell.

Reminder: Please write out the first thing that comes into your mind; don't think about the questions too much.

The iliopsoas, Quads, and Low-Back Questions

What is your favorite way to move?

What pleases you in your life?

What is the overall state of health of your pelvic bowl?

What is the state of health of your lower back? Painful or no pain?

What is your relationship to money?

What do you do when confronted with change?

What are your feelings used for?

What emotion or emotions do you normally feel?

What is your level of emotional literacy on a scale from 1-10? (1) meaning I don't understand my feelings at all; (10) meaning I know how to manage my emotions.

What is your awareness level of others' feelings on a scale from 1-10? (1) I don't understand other people's feelings at all. (10) I totally merge with others who are emoting and feel their feelings.

Spend a Moment with Your Iliopsoas, Quads, and Low-Back
What is your low-back trying to say to you?

What are you afraid of?

Low-Back Standing, Walking, and Sitting Questions
Does your sacrum (the triangular bone at the back of your pelvis) move up as the front of your pelvis tips down?

Does your sacrum root down and the front of your pelvic bowl tilt up?

Does one hip push forward more than the other hip?

Is one hip bone lifted up more than the other?

Is your lower back in neutral – meaning that you have a slight curve in your lower back and the front of your pelvis is pulled slightly up, with both hips balanced and even?

Low-Back Trauma Questions
What pain do you have in your lower back? Describe it in detail.

What is stressing you out?

The Common Challenges of the Low-Back
Sacroiliac (SI) joint issues - The sacroiliac (SI) joints are held together by ligaments and tendons. When you have a hypermobile pelvis, the sacrum can pop out of joint from the sacral ligaments

and tendons becoming overstretched. Unfortunately, once the ligaments and tendons are overstretched in the sacral area, you will always have to work to keep them in.

Do you have pain on one side of your low-back more than the other? (It could be caused by a dislocated SI joint).

Herniated discs, bulging discs, and degenerative disc disease are all caused by compression in the lower back. The energetic meaning behind this compression is fear.

What lower back issues do you have?

Broken pelvic bowl - usually happens in older women due to osteoporosis.

What is the state of health of your pelvis and hip bones?

Look your answers over and consider the main things that you learned about yourself from doing this questionnaire. What did you learn? Jot down your answers.

Now, let's get your low-back open!

The Low-Back Movement Practice

You'll need your yoga mat, Noodle Ball, and chair.

A reminder:

- Do what you can. If something is too challenging, don't do it and make a note in the book, as it was designed as a workbook.
- Make a note of the exercises and practices that have the greatest impact on you.
- Remember the *Haaaa* Breath. Use it while you do each practice.

Ball Work – The Low-Back

Noodle Ball Up Your Spine

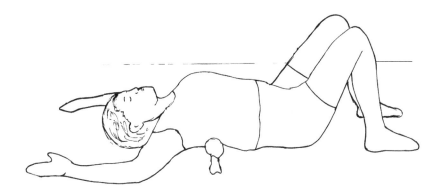

Place the Noodle Ball horizontally into your mid-butt cheeks. Rock side to side and slowly move up and into your low-back and mid-back, keeping your knees bent. Take your arms overhead as you move into your heart space. Continue moving up until the Noodle Ball falls off your shoulders.

Stretches - Iliopsoas, Quads, and Low-Back

Hug Your Knees –

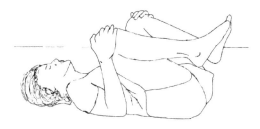

Lie on your back and bring your knees to your chest. Gently hug your knees and breathe deeply in and out of your belly. Feel your knees dropping into your body as you exhale and move away from your body as you inhale. Rest here feeling the gentle rocking motion.

When ready, make circles slowly going in both directions. You can also rock gently from side to side. Breathe as you rock and/or circle. **This pose can bring you a tremendous amount of relief from low-back pain.**

Iliopsoas Quad Opener –

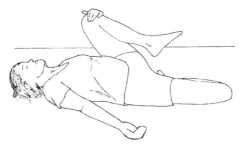

From lying down, bring your knees to your chest. On an exhalation, bring your left foot to the floor, keeping your right knee into your chest. Walk your left foot to the right. Drop your left knee to the floor as you pull your left heel into the center of your right butt cheek with your right hand. Hold, breathe, and let go of fear.

Switch sides and do the same thing on the other side.

Lying Squat –

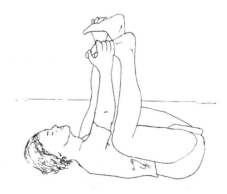

Bring both knees to your chest, pause, and come into a lying squat by holding the balls of both feet with your hands and drawing your knees to the outer edge of your body. Use a strap on the balls of your feet if necessary. Your heels move away from your buttocks and feet toward your head. Breathe, allowing the body to move on the waves of the breath.

All Fours –

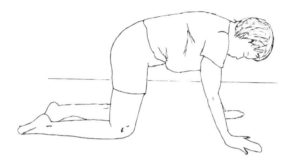

Come onto all fours by bringing your knees under your hips and your hands under your shoulders on all fours. Bring your ribs up and in toward your pelvis, roll your inner arms out, and squeeze your scapula together keeping a long lower back. From there, you can move your head and neck around and circle your hips in both directions.

Lunge –

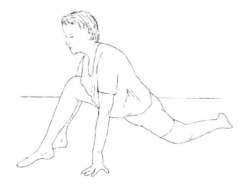

From all fours, step your right leg forward into a lunge. Walk the right foot as far forward as possible. Press your back foot into the earth and drop your pelvis down and forward.

Roll the inner arms out and on each exhale drop your tail and inhale open your heart. Use a block if it's difficult to get your hands to the floor. On an exhale, pull your right knee into your chest and turn your chest to your right knee. Hold and breathe, dropping your tail down on each exhalation.

Switch sides when ready by backing up your bottom and stepping back to all fours and do the same thing on the other side.

Lunge Dropping To Elbows –

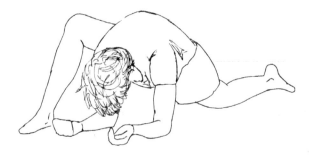

From all fours, step your right leg forward and walk your right foot as far forward as it will go. Drop your tail down and forward. Use a block if you have trouble bringing your hands to the floor. Hold and breathe.

Take your hands to the inside of your right foot. Walk your right foot further forward if you can. When ready, exhale and bend your elbows, placing them on the floor without letting your pelvis fall forward. Feel the stretch deep in your inner upper leg. If you can't do this, stay up on your hands or place your hands on a block. Hold and breathe.

When ready to come out, back your bottom up and step your front foot back. Come to all fours, switch sides, and do the same thing on the other side.

This releases the upper inner quad muscles.

Strengthening - The Quads, Iliopsoas, and Low-Back

Down Dog –

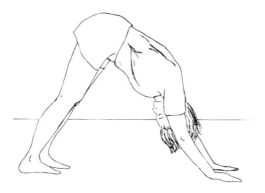

Go back to all fours with hands under shoulders, knees under hips, ribs up and in. Roll your inner arms out as you squeeze your shoulder blades together.

Exhale, lift your knees, and come up to Down Dog, pressing your heels to (or toward) the floor. Hold and breathe for about two minutes.

Down Dog With The Leg Back –

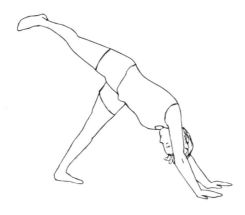

From Down Dog, bring your right leg straight back behind you, lift your right hip to the sky, and bring your straight strong right leg back behind you. Hold and breathe. When ready, switch sides and do the same thing on the other side. Let go of fear.

Standing Posture –

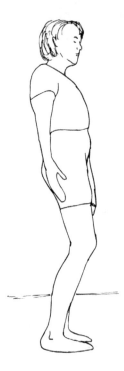

Stand with your feet inner hip-width apart, lined up from the inside of your hip bones. Press into the outer edge of your heels, lift and spread your toes, then set them down gently on the earth without gripping. Feel your legs ground.

Allow your sacrum and tail to drop down and your ribs to snap in and down toward your pelvis. Roll your inner arms out and squeeze your scapula together, forming back cleavage. Breathe in and out of your open heart and allow your head to rest on top of your spine.

Standing Yoga Nidra –

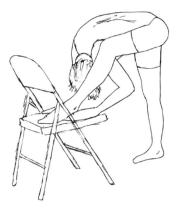

Stand in front of a chair in your new low-back posture. Take your right foot up on the chair, bend forward and attempt to tuck your right shoulder under your right knee. Hold and breathe. Come out, switch sides, and do the same thing on the other side.

Forward Fold –

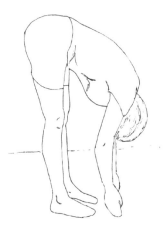

From standing, on an exhalation, drop forward into a standing forward bend. Allow your upper body to be loose and free, your legs to ground down, your knees slightly bent and your feet to connect deeply to the earth. Push into the outer edge of your heels and spread your toes wide apart. Breathe and hold.

Child's Pose –

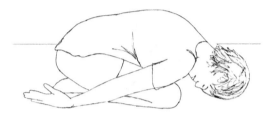

From all fours, bring your bottom back to rest on your heels. If your knees hurt, don't go back to the heels.

Allow your head to come to the floor, arms alongside your body, or overhead. Let go and breathe and feel what you've done in this practice.

Hug Your Knees –

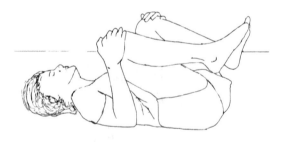

Lie on your back and bring your knees to your chest. Gently hug your knees and breathe deeply in and out of your belly. Feel your knees dropping into your body as you exhale and move away from your body as you inhale. Rest here feeling the gentle rocking motion.

When ready, make circles slowly going in both directions. You can also rock gently from side to side. Breathe as you rock and/

or circle. **This pose can bring you a tremendous amount of relief from low-back pain.**

Yoga Nidra –

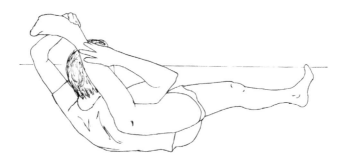

From Hug your Knees, take your right foot into your right hand and drop your right knee to the outer edge of your body. Pull your right foot toward your head as you straighten your left leg keeping your left heel off the floor.

Place your left hand on your right heel. Bring your right arm to the inside of your right leg, round up, lift your head and bring your right knee over your right shoulder. If you can, bring your foot behind your head. If your foot doesn't go behind your head, place a block behind your head. Hold and breathe. Switch sides and do the same thing on the other side.

This pose lengthens your low-back and helps your sacrum go back into alignment.

Rest –

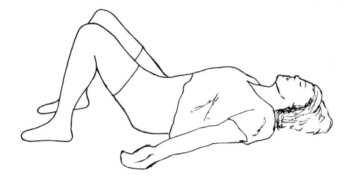

Lie on your back with your knees bent and your feet resting on the floor. Feel your lower back resting on the earth and breathe in and out of your pelvic bowl. Roll your inner arms out and rest them on the floor with your palms facing up. Soften your shoulders, move your head gently from side to side and if your chin falls away from your chest, place a pillow behind your head. Go into stillness and feel your body breathing.

Chapter 13 - Power Your Core and Strengthen the Belly

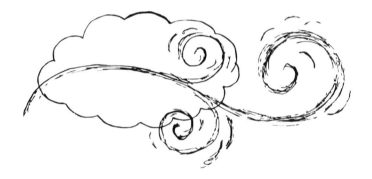

Are you looking for me? I am in the next seat.
My shoulder is against yours.
You will not find me in stupas, not in Indian shrine rooms,
nor in synagogues, nor in cathedrals:
not in masses, nor in kirtans, not in legs winding around your
own neck, nor in eating nothing but vegetables.
When you really look for me, you will see me instantly—
you will find me in the tiniest house of time.
Kabir says: Student, tell me what is God?
He is the breath inside the breath.

Kabir

Breathing Lessons

The diaphragm is the breathing muscle of the body. It is shaped like a mushroom and sits at the floor of the heart and lungs and on the ceiling of the belly.

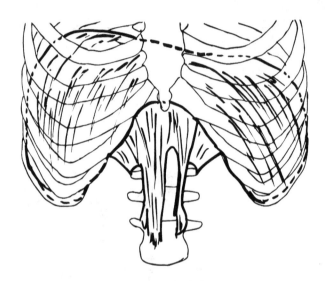

Your diaphragm was designed to pull the breath in by moving down toward the belly with each inhalation. The diaphragm pushes the breath out by moving up toward the heart and lungs with each exhalation.

Most of us have breath-holding patterns that don't allow us to fully, deeply, and completely take the breath in and out of our bodies. In fact, very few people use their diaphragm to breathe.

This means the majority of us need breathing lessons. To help you understand how to fully diaphragmatically breathe, I'll first dive into the two most common breath-holding patterns. They are:

Breathing with the secondary breathing muscles, the shoulders and neck, instead of the diaphragm. The diaphragm is stuck and doesn't move to pull the breath in and out of the body.

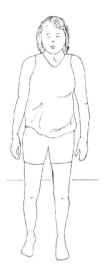

This breathing pattern causes anxiety, as the secondary breathing muscles are there to give us that extra boost of breath when something is chasing us and we need to move quickly. If we primarily breathe with our neck and shoulder muscles, the nervous system thinks that we are perpetually under attack.

Reverse breathing is when the diaphragm moves in the opposite direction it was meant to.

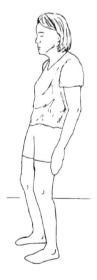

In reverse breathing, the diaphragm moves up with each inhalation and down with each exhalation. This breathing pattern causes confusion and disorientation, as the body's very life force, the breath, is moving in and out of the body in the opposite direction it was designed to move.

Now that we've explored the two most common breath-holding patterns, let's dive into how to breathe correctly!

Full Diaphragmatic Breathing Lessons

Lie on your back with your knees bent. If your chin lifts up toward the ceiling, place a small pillow behind your head so that your chin drops down and in toward your body. Relax and become aware of your breath moving in and out of your body.

Place your hands on your belly.

Breathe in and see if you can feel your belly rising up as the diaphragm moves and pushes your belly contents toward your pelvis and out in front of you.

Breathe out and feel your belly drop down and toward your heart as your diaphragm moves up.

Keep breathing like this and see if you can feel the expansion of the belly as you inhale and the belly dropping down and back as you exhale.

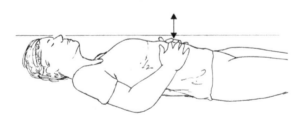

If you do feel these movements in your belly, congratulations!! You are breathing using your diaphragm.

If you don't feel your belly moving up and out with each inhalation and back down and up with each exhalation, don't worry. You can learn to breathe like this by practicing and adding a deep massage of the diaphragm at the end of each exhalation.

Diaphragm massage – To do this, lie back down with your knees bent. If your chin lifts toward the ceiling, place a small pillow behind your head so that your chin drops down and in toward your body. Relax and feel yourself breathing.

Place your hands on your belly.

Breathe in and see if you can feel your belly rising up as the diaphragm moves down and pushes your belly contents down and out. Breathe out saying, "*Haaaa.*" As you come to the bottom of your exhalation, dig your fingers deep under your rib cage and massage by pressing your fingers in and up. Keep breathing like this and massaging under your ribs. Over time this stimulation will begin to break up the stuck fascia that is holding the diaphragm muscle in its holding pattern.

The Greatest Challenge Worksheet

We all face numerous life challenges that can limit our thinking, trigger negative responses, cause self-sabotage, and lead us to compromise ourselves; all of which will cause us stress, which leads to low-back pain!!

Knowing what our life challenges are is the first step in converting them into our purpose, which allows us to take our power back. Once in our power, we can release stress.

Scan the Life Challenges list below and check off any items that grab your attention. Be open and receptive and your intuition will flag items that deserve consideration.

Check the box for any life challenges that 'resonate' with you.

Common Life Challenges

- abandonment
- absentmindedness

- abuse
- accidents
- accusing
- acting the clown
- addictions
- aggression
- always being with people
- ambition
- analyzing
- anger
- anxiety
- arguing
- arrogance
- attachment
- avoidance
- being judgmental
- being opinionated
- being reactive
- being scattered
- being too emotional
- being ungrounded
- blaming
- blind devotion
- boredom
- bossiness
- busyness
- boredom
- carelessness
- codependency
- complaining
- compromise
- compulsion
- conflict
- confusion
- control

- cowardice
- criticism
- cruelty
- cynicism
- deceitfulness
- deception
- defensiveness
- defiance
- denial
- dependency
- depression
- deviousness
- discounting
- dishonesty
- disorder
- disoriented
- dominance
- doubt
- drama
- dreaming
- egotism
- emotions
- envy
- escape
- exaggeration
- excessive focus on others
- excuses
- extremism
- failure
- fantasizing
- faulty beliefs
- fears
- feeling needy
- fixed ideas
- focusing on the past

- foolishness
- forgetfulness
- frustration
- futility
- future thinking
- glamour
- greed
- guilt
- hate
- hopelessness
- humorlessness
- humor
- ignorance
- ignoring
- illness
- illusions
- impatience
- impractical
- impulsiveness
- inaccuracy
- indecision
- indifference
- inertia
- inflexible character
- injury
- insecurity
- insensitivity
- intellectualization
- intolerance
- isolation
- jealousy
- judging
- justifying limitations
- lack of commitment
- lack of confidence

- lack of creativity
- lack of discipline
- lack of energy
- lack of purpose
- lack of trust
- laughing it off
- laziness
- living in the past
- loneliness
- low energy
- lying
- malnutrition
- manipulation
- martyrdom
- materialism
- mediocrity
- minimizing
- moodiness
- narrowness
- needing to please others
- negativity
- no fun
- non-supportive habits
- numbness
- obsessions
- opportunism
- over-eating
- over-exercising
- over-spending
- overwhelm
- over-working
- pain
- perfectionism
- phobias
- poor health

- poor self-esteem
- possessiveness
- poverty mentality
- prejudice
- pride
- procrastination
- rationalization
- rebellion
- repression
- resentment
- resistance
- ridicule
- rudeness
- running away
- sadness
- sarcasm
- seeking approval
- self-obsession
- self-centeredness
- self-deception
- selfishness
- self-pity
- self-sabotaging
- shame
- shyness
- sleep
- solitude
- status
- stress
- stubbornness
- suffering
- timidity
- unexpressed emotions
- vacillating

- vanity
- violence
- withdrawing
- worrying

Now, go back to those boxes that you've checked and choose the top five Life Challenges for further exploration.

Sit with these five top choices and see if they have a theme. For instance, if my top five choices were abandonment, addictions, co-dependence, excessive focus on others, and running away, I have a theme of leaving myself.

I may then narrow down my greatest challenge by putting the top themes together and ending up with a life challenge statement similar to this —

Abandoning myself through codependent addictive relation-ships, where I excessively focus on others until I can't take it anymore and I run away.

How to Face and Overcome Your Greatest Challenge to Fulfill Your Life's Purpose

You came to life on this earth to overcome your greatest challenge. That is the reason you are here.

We remain in the dark and feel confused and stressed when we think that our purpose is something like healing other people or working to achieve world peace. These are lofty goals, but they are NOT your purpose.

Again — YOU came here to overcome the thing that challenges you most in this life.

You've already defined that challenge. Here's my greatest challenge as an example:

My greatest life challenge is focusing all of my attention on the care of others: their physical well-being, their feelings, and their lives in general, to the detriment of my own health, goals, dreams, and passions.

1. What is your greatest challenge? Write it down here:

Your life challenge can cause you pain or harm. For example, my pain is: When I take care of others, I lose myself and I get off-balance. From that off-balance place, I can get tired, cranky, and be less than loving toward others in my life. I also can build walls around people who I perceive have *taken too much from me.*

2. What pain or harm does your life's challenge create for you?

Are you ready to leave that pain behind for good? Once you know your challenge and begin to work your way toward its opposite – your purpose – you are on the right path. You can feel it and relax into knowing why you are here. I call this path your spiritual path. Your work is to focus all your energy toward the fulfillment of your purpose.

3. What is the opposite of your life's challenge?

The opposite of your life's challenge is your purpose. My challenge is focusing on others more than myself. So, my purpose is to focus on myself. To take care of myself. I like to say, *I'm here to love myself.*

When I am working on taking care of myself, I am on my spiritual path. When I leave my own needs behind and focus too much on others, I've turned away from my purpose and backed off from my spiritual path.

So, what is the opposite of your life's challenge?

4. It is your purpose ... What is that? Write it down.
My life's purpose is ...

5. Make your life's purpose your focus by writing it down and putting up reminders to yourself in places you will see it often,

like on your bathroom mirror, your car's steering wheel, or your computer.

I write on sticky notes — *Michelle, you are here to take care of yourself and learn to love YOU!*

Now, you might be thinking, it's good to take care of others. Yes, I agree, but not when you sacrifice yourself to do so. You may also be thinking, to focus so much on yourself is selfish. That may be true – if your life's challenge is focusing on yourself at the cost of others.

What I'm getting at is that for me to come into balance, I must walk away from my life's challenge of focusing on others and toward its opposite – focusing on myself. That is my purpose. I won't ever become selfish, because it is ingrained in my being to take care of others. I just need to take care of myself first; to think of myself more often. To achieve this, I must continuously work to focus on loving myself. Then I'll be in balance.

Once YOU know your purpose…

6. When confronted with a choice, ask yourself: Does this choice take me toward my life's purpose or take me away from my life's purpose?

It is my commitment to choose to love myself. The more I do this, the better I get at it. The more I choose myself, the closer I come to fulfilling my life's purpose.

And the side benefit is that I release stress, come into balance, and take better care of myself. I'm also happier and have less low-back pain.

7. Do you want to experience more happiness in your life?

8. Will you commit yourself to focusing on fulfilling your life's purpose?

I'm sure you will! See you on the path walking toward your life's purpose!

Inquiry Questions: The Belly

These questions are designed to get you thinking beyond the physical manifestation of your low-back pain.

The belly is your power center. When the belly is strong and open, you are living from your value system as you fulfill your life's purpose.

Reminder: Please write out the first thing that comes into your mind; don't think about the questions too much.

The Belly Questions

What is your definition of power?

What makes you feel like a victim?

What causes you to become aggressive?

What do you do to empower yourself?

What areas in your life do you take action?

What areas in your life are you stuck?

What is your soul's truth?

What does your personality show the world?

What feeling do you have about moving from the safety of the known into the unknown?

What is the change that you wish to see in the world?

What do you take responsibility for in your life?

What do you blame others for in your life?

What mistakes are okay for you to make?

What addictions do you have?

What control do you have over yourself?

What reaction do you have toward authority?

What do you resist?

Spend a Moment with Your Belly
Look at your belly —

What amount of excessive fat do you carry around your belly?

What core strength do you have?

What do your ribs do? Flare out, or drop in toward your body and down toward your pelvis?

Belly Trauma Questions
What causes your stomach to hurt? For example, spicy food, fighting with a loved one, public speaking, or standing up for yourself.

What causes you to doubt your self-worth?

Check your answers and consider the main things that you learned about yourself from doing this questionnaire. What did you learn? Jot down your answers.

Now, we will move on to discovering our core values.

Core Values

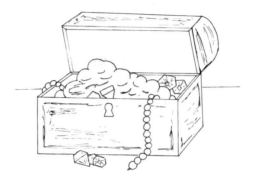

Living from your value system is key to reducing stress and releasing low-back pain. When we don't live from what is most valuable to us, our whole system goes haywire, and we are guaranteed to live in a state of stress and ultimately experience low-back pain.

Fortunately, it is easy to discover what is most important to you. You were born with certain innate values. Life experiences and the influence of other people may have shifted you away from these core values, but it is never too late to claim them and live from your truth.

Below is a list of common core values. This list is not all-inclusive, but it will give you a good idea of various personal values. Select your top three core values from the list below.

Here's how to do that — Check every value that appeals to you. When you are done, rank the values and choose your top three.

Core Values List

- Authenticity
- Achievement
- Adventure
- Authority
- Autonomy
- Balance
- Beauty
- Boldness

- Compassion
- Challenge
- Citizenship
- Community
- Competency
- Communication
- Contribution
- Creativity
- Curiosity
- Determination
- Fairness
- Faith
- Fame
- Friendships
- Fun
- Growth
- Happiness
- Health
- Honesty
- Humor
- Influence
- Inner Harmony
- Justice
- Kindness
- Knowledge
- Leadership
- Learning
- Love
- Loyalty
- Meaningful Work
- Openness
- Optimism
- Peace
- Pleasure
- Poise

- Popularity
- Recognition
- Religion
- Reputation
- Respect
- Responsibility
- Security
- Self-Respect
- Service
- Spirituality
- Stability
- Success
- Status
- Trustworthiness
- Wealth
- Wisdom

Once you've selected your three top values, write a brief sentence to describe your values.

For example —

1. The value of Growth - To continue to do my personal work to grow into the best person I can be.
2. The value of Communication - To always show up for all conversations, even the tough ones, using two tools. Council (which is the way the indigenous people worked things out, by sitting in a circle and using a talking stick to honor the person speaking by listening); and Non-Violent Communication (NVC) developed by Marshall Rosenberg. NVC is a way to connect and communicate with ourselves and others from the heart).
3. The value of Health - To move and eat every day in a way that keeps my body happy.

Write out your top three values and place them somewhere you'll see them every day. Once you are consciously aware and reminded of your core values, it becomes easier to make sure that every choice you make aligns with them. And that means less stress in your low-back and in your life!

The Belly Movement Practice

You'll need your yoga mat, softball-sized ball, Noodle Ball, and wall space.

A reminder:

- Do what you can. If something is too challenging, don't do it and make a note in the book, as it was designed as a workbook.
- Make a note of the exercises and practices that have the greatest impact on you.
- Remember the *Haaaa* Breath. Use it while you do each practice.

Ball Work – Belly

Ball From Your Iliopsoas into Your Psoas –

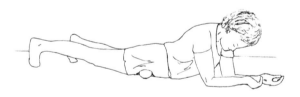

Place the ball beside your right hip bone. Roll into your pubic bone and back to your hip bone, opening your iliopsoas. Slowly roll up and around the pelvic rim, coming to the outer edge of your belly, which is where you will feel your psoas. Roll slightly in toward your belly and back out to the outer edge of your body, back and forth, and up to the edge of your floating ribs. Hold there and breathe.

Follow the outer edge of the ribs, breathing into the ball as you inhale and exhale allowing the ball to fall into you. Keep going until you come to the V of the ribs. Pause and inhale and exhale here for a couple of breaths.

Follow the left outer edge of the ribs to the outer edge of your belly connecting to your left psoas. Continue along the left edge of your belly to the pelvic rim, and to the inside of your left hip bone. Here, rock into your pubic bone and back to your hip bone releasing your iliopsoas.

Noodle Ball up your spine –

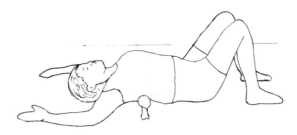

Place the Noodle Ball horizontally into your mid-butt cheeks. Rock side to side and slowly move up and into your low-back and mid-back, keeping your knees bent. Take your arms overhead as you move into your heart space. Continue moving up until the Noodle Ball falls off your shoulders.

Stretches – Belly

Clock Pose –

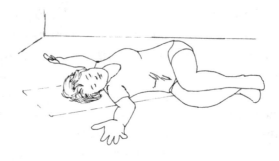

Lie on your back with your knees to your chest. Bring your knees up and into your chest and keep them there as you roll over onto your right side. Take your arms out even with your shoulders, and on an exhale bring your left arm overhead, keeping your fingertips on the floor. Inhale your arm back and exhale overhead three times, then hold and breathe in love!

Come out and lie on your side, then roll onto your back. Rest, switch sides, and do the same thing on the other side.

Strengtheners – Belly

Belly strengthener at the wall –

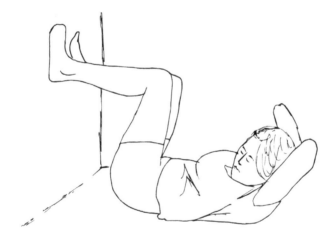

Lie on your back and put your feet on the wall at a right angle. Make sure your feet are lined up with your inner legs. Press into the outer edges of your heels as you lift your big toes. Feel the length of your low-back against the floor.

Put your right hand behind your left shoulder and your left hand behind your right shoulder, cradling your head. Breathe in and out of your belly. On an exhale, lift up, taking your right elbow toward your left knee. Hold and breathe for as long as you can. Come down on an exhale, and rest.

Switch sides by lifting up on an exhale and taking your left elbow toward your right knee. Hold and breathe as long as you can. Come down on an exhale, and rest. Do it as many times as you are comfortable.

Squats –

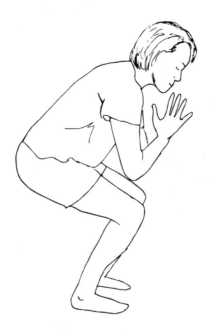

From standing, take your feet inner hip-width apart (or outer hip-width apart if you don't practice squats). Press into the outer edges of your heels, making sure your feet are facing straight ahead without ducking or pigeon-toeing.

Drop your tail, and take your ribs in and down toward your pelvic bowl. Roll your inner arms out and squeeze your shoulder blades together.

Exhale, bend your knees as far as you can — DO NOT go into knee pain!

Exhale, come down into a squat, inhale back up and continue. Build up to doing 50 squats a day.

Anatomy of Your Abdominals, Diaphragm and Erectors

The Diaphragm

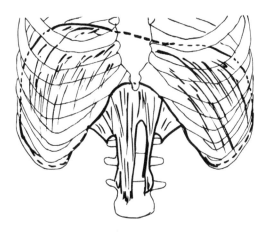

Your diaphragm is the principal breathing muscle.

Learning to fully breathe using the diaphragm and relaxing the shoulders allows your whole body to relax and ride on the waves of the breath as it moves in and out of your body.

The diaphragm also massages our internal organs: it moves down as we breathe in, pushing the belly contents out. The diaphragm is an extra pump for the heart. As we breathe out, the diaphragm moves up and pushes out the air from the lungs and bumps into the heart.

To fully breathe, our bellies must be free to expand as we inhale and to contract as we exhale.

Most women were taught to hold their bellies in, in order to have a flat stomach. This only creates a weak core as the low-back is forced to do the work of the abdominals — causing back pain!!

The Abdominals

In the Belly Movement Practices, you'll strengthen the muscles of the belly, which are the abdominals.

The abdominals consist of **four separate muscles.**

Here is a drawing that shows where each one is located:

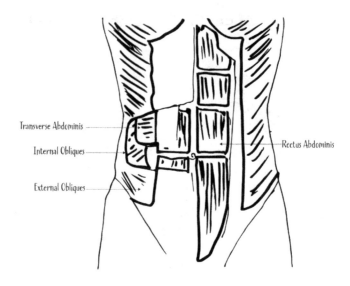

Together, these muscles will impact your core stability, strength, and your posture.

Rectus Abdominis Muscle

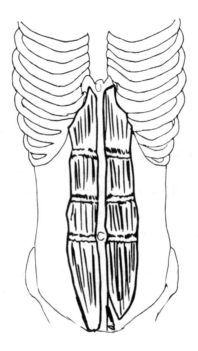

When people refer to a "six-pack," this is the muscle that they are talking about. The rectus abdominis is positioned between the ribs and the pubic bone at the front of the pelvis and is made up of eight distinct muscles.

When the muscle contracts, these muscle bellies are visible. If the level of body fat is low enough, it will create that "six-pack" look.

The rectus abdominis is essential for maintaining good posture and is primarily responsible for flexing the lumbar spine (the movement of a sit-up or a crunch).

This muscle can be worked out in two different ways: by either bringing the chest towards the pelvis (as with a crunch) or by bringing the pelvis towards the chest (as with a leg raise).

This type of exercise is what people mean when they say they're working their "upper"' or "lower" abs.

Finally, the rectus abdominis also helps to regulate breathing and protects your internal organs by creating intra-abdominal pressure.

External Obliques

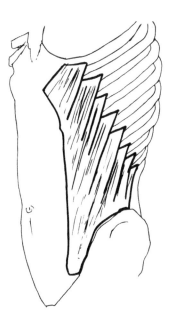

The external oblique muscles are two distinct sets of oblique muscles: your external obliques and your internal obliques.

Your external obliques sit on either side of your rectus abdominis and are the largest of your abdominal muscles.

External obliques allow the trunk of your body to twist. Twisting is controlled by the external oblique muscle on the opposite side of the direction that you're twisting.

For instance, if you are twisting to the left, you are using your right external oblique.

The external obliques also help with your overall posture, pulling your chest downwards and protecting your organs by creating intra-abdominal pressure (just as with the rectus abdominis).

Internal Obliques

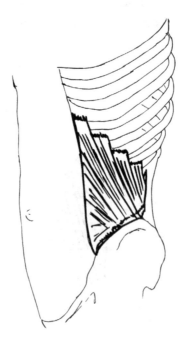

Internal oblique muscles are the opposite of the external oblique.

They are located directly below the rectus abdominis and sit just inside your hip bones.

The internal obliques are also responsible for twisting and turning, but they control the other side of the movement.

For example, when you twist to the right, you are contracting both your *right* internal oblique and your *left* external oblique at the same time.

Since they control the movement on the same side of your body, internal obliques are sometimes referred to as "same-side rotators."

Transverse Abdominis

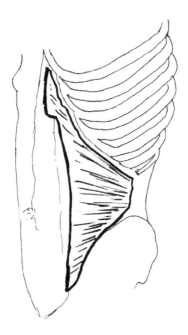

The transverse abdominis muscle is a very important muscle, integral to holding your entire abdominal structure together.

The transverse abdominis is the 'deepest' of your ab muscles, located underneath your rectus abdominis and obliques.

Even though you'll never see this muscle visually, it is key to maintaining a functionally strong core and creating large amounts of stabilizing internal abdominal pressure.

The Erectors

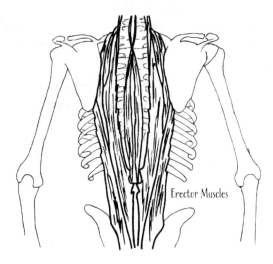

Erector Muscles

The erector spinae muscles are a group of long muscles that originate near the sacrum and extend vertically up the length of the back. The erector spinae muscles lie on each side of the vertebral column and extend alongside the lumbar, thoracic, and cervical sections of the spine.

The erector spinae muscles function to straighten the back and allow for side-to-side rotation. An injury or strain to these muscles may cause back spasms and pain.

A Pain-Free Low-Back Story –

Pamela found me a couple of months after her hip replacement surgery because her low-back continued to hurt on the left side. She'd had surgery to help alleviate this pain.

After her low-back assessment, I diagnosed Pamela with a dislocated left sacroiliac joint that was out of place. I showed her the daily practice that she needed to do, which included lengthening her back, putting her sacrum back in place, and strengthening her core.

Pamela said: *I had no idea my sacroiliac (SI) joint was out of place. I've had pain there for years, yet no one in the medical community noticed my SI joint was dislocated. I'm wondering if I really needed that hip replacement. Doing the core work made me realize how weak my abdominals were. With the practices from Michelle, I now can keep my SI joint in place, which takes away my low-back pain and allows me to take walks and enjoy life again.*

Chapter 14 – Releasing Sciatica

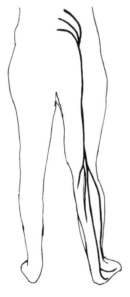

Kali, be with us
Violence, destruction, receive our homage.
Help us to bring darkness into the light,
To lift out the pain, the anger,
Where it can be seen for what it is –
The balance-wheel for our vulnerable, aching love.
May Sarton

So many of us with low-back pain have sciatica. Sciatica is nerve pain running from the butt cheek down into the leg and sometimes down to the foot. It is caused by a pinch or grab of the nerve somewhere along its pathway from the sacrum into the butt cheek, through or alongside the piriformis, and down into the leg.

Sciatica can be tricky to release because the nerve often gets pinched by a bundle of scar tissue, and once pinched an indent might remain. Kind of like when you put your fingernail into a piece of styrofoam. The good thing about a sciatic nerve indent is that it can be healed.

The first step in releasing sciatica is to let go of the piriformis tension with myofascial release ball work. The second step is to stretch the piriformis. I'll show you how to do this both lying down and standing up.

Remember that releasing the pinch of the sciatic nerve doesn't always bring instant relief. You'll have to keep doing this practice consistently to keep the press of the muscle off the nerve, and the indent may take some time to heal.

To complicate matters even more, you may have to locate the mass of scar tissue that is pinching and pulling on the nerve and work that out. This mass is usually found in the butt cheek (piriformis) on the side where you experience sciatica.

Lying Sciatica Release Practice
You'll need your yoga mat and softball-sized ball.

Ball Work – Sciatica

Ball in Your Butt Cheek –

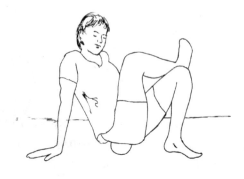

Lie down or sit up with a softball-sized ball in your right butt cheek. Place your right ankle on your left knee. Roll around seeking knots of tension. Stay on the knots and move back and forth over them, breathing out control of *others*.

Switch sides after two minutes and place the ball in your left butt cheek, with your left ankle on your right knee. Roll around seeking knots of tension. Stay on the knots and move back and forth over them, breathing out control of *yourself*.

Ball in the side of your butt cheek –

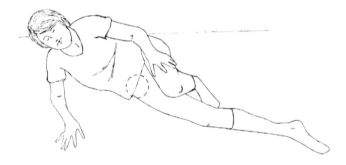

Roll to your side and place a softball-sized ball in the indent of your butt cheek. Straighten your bottom leg. Move the ball up and down in the C-like curve.

Stretches – Sciatica

Butt Cheek Stretch –

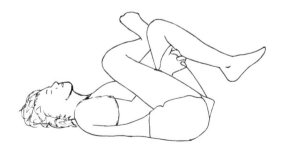

Lie on your back and place your right ankle on your left knee. Place your hands on the back of your left thigh and draw your left knee toward your chest. Find your edge (the end of your comfort zone; as far as you can go), then hold and breathe. Let go of control of your outer world and breathe in acceptance of whatever comes your way.

When ready, switch sides and place the left ankle on the right knee. On this side breathe out letting go of control of yourself and breathe in acceptance.

Standing Sciatica Release Practice
You'll need wall space and a softball-sized ball.

Ball Work – Sciatica

A Ball into Your Butt Cheek at the Wall –

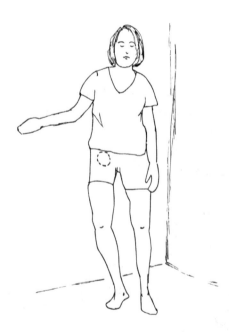

Place a softball-sized ball into the butt cheek on the side where you experience sciatica. Roll around seeking the knots of tension and wiggle back and forth on them. You can turn to your side and dig into the C-like indent of the butt cheek as well.

Stretches – Sciatica

Standing Butt Cheek Stretch –

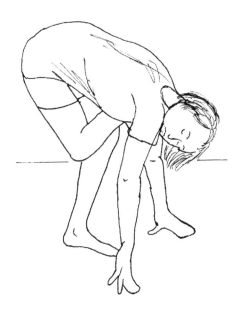

Stand next to a wall for balance. Stand into the leg that is not experiencing sciatica pain and take the ankle of the leg that is experiencing sciatica onto the knee of the standing leg.

Bend the standing leg as you fall forward, bringing your hands to the floor (or to a chair seat or to the wall).

Find your edge (the end of your comfort zone; as far as you can go) by bending the standing leg as much as you can and holding and breathing for two minutes. Breathe out control and breathe in acceptance.

Do this practice as many times a day as you can. The more you release the piriformis, the quicker your sciatica will let go.

A Pain-Free Low-Back Story –

Robin loved to golf and had moved to Florida so that she could play year-round. She sought help from me when her low-back and sciatica pain became so severe that it prevented her from golfing.

Robin saw doctors, physical therapists, and chiropractors without a reduction in pain. She also tried acupuncture and Pilates to see if they would ease her pain, but nothing changed.

That's when I met Robin. After assessing Robin's posture, I could see she had a tight left piriformis (control) muscle. We began to work on releasing that tight, stuck muscle, and Robin's low-back pain eased. Her sciatica went away and Robin went back to playing golf.

A couple of months later Robin went golfing as usual, but that day she twisted funny and her sciatica immediately came back. She'd been keeping up her practice but not every day. She immediately got back to her daily practice, got herself out of pain, and has kept the pain away for almost a year now.

Robin shares: *I was in so much pain in my low-back and down my left leg that I had to give up my golf game. I love to golf, so I quickly got on it and saw my doctor who recommended physical therapy. All that did was make the pain worse, so I tried seeing a chiropractor, getting acupuncture, and even joining a Pilates class. Nothing helped.*

Then I met Michelle. She was the first person to look at my posture and recognized right away what the problem was. I had a tight left butt cheek and a weak core. I saw results right away and was soon back to playing golf.

When the pain came back I immediately knew what to do and I got myself right back out of pain. I now never miss doing my daily practice.

Chapter 15 – Releasing Sacroiliac Joint Problems

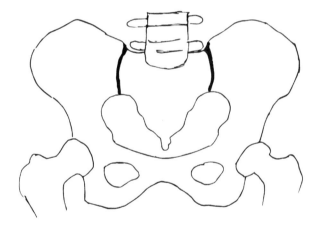

You and I were a natural disaster.
And just like most eruptions,
We erupted when it was least expected.
Maybe now, I can cool.
I can stabilize and reform.
You can finally get the stability you need.
J.R. Falk

A common low-back issue that often goes undiagnosed by the standard medical community is sacroiliac (SI) joint issues. The SI joints are located on either side of the sacrum. They can slip out of joint by the muscular imbalances most of us have around our pelvic bowl or low-back.

How do you know you have an SI joint issue?
You'll have pain in the SI joint. It may be swollen and sticking out more than the other side. SI joint pain usually presents as a constant ache, although it can be a sharp pain when you try to move when the SI joint is out.

Unfortunately, once an SI joint goes out it means the ligaments and tendons that hold it in place are overstretched, so it can easily go out again.

I know all about SI joint challenges. I have an SI joint that goes out of alignment and it was misdiagnosed for years. For some reason, doctors, physical therapists, and even chiropractors don't pay attention to the SI Joint. Because of this, I lived in pain with an SI joint out of alignment for years!

Fortunately for you, I figured out a way to get the SI joint back in place and have it stay in place. Your daily practice is designed to get your low-back and pelvic bowl into alignment and your core strengthened, so that your SI joint will have a better chance of staying where it belongs!

Lying SI Joint Practice
You'll need your yoga mat and softball-sized ball.

Ball in Your SI joint –

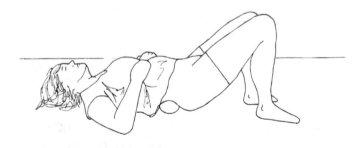

Lie down and place a ball right on the SI joint on the side that hurts. It will feel like you are on a swollen, often painful bump. Keep the ball here while you breathe slowly in and out for about thirty seconds. Move down on that same side to midway between the top of the sacrum and the tail, staying on the outer edge of the sacrum. Hold again for thirty seconds. Then move down to just above your deep gluteal cleft (butt crack), the bottom of the sacrum, and hold again for thirty seconds.

Hug Your Knees –

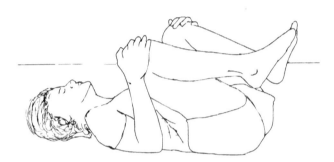

Lie on your back and bring your knees to your chest. Gently hug your knees and breathe deeply in and out of your belly. Feel your knees dropping into your body as you exhale, and moving away from your body as you inhale. Rest here feeling the gentle rocking motion.

When ready, make circles slowly going in both directions. You can also rock gently from side to side. Breathe as you rock and/or circle. **This pose can bring you a tremendous amount of relief from low-back pain.**

Half Lying Squat –

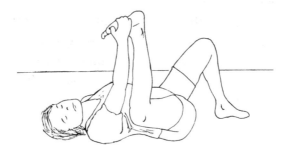

Lie on your back. On the same side the sacrum is out, take hold of that foot and pull that foot toward your head as the knee drops toward the floor. Drop the opposite foot to the floor. If you can, round up and place that foot behind your head taking Yoga Nidra (see below). Hold and breathe on your edge (the end of your comfort zone; as far as you can go) for two minutes.

Yoga Nidra –

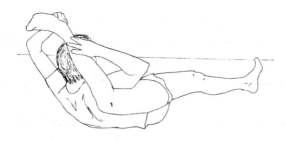

From Hug your Knees, take your right foot into your right hand and drop your right knee to the outer edge of your body. Pull your right foot toward your head as you straighten your left leg keeping your left heel off the floor.

Place your left hand on your right heel. Bring your right arm to the inside of your right leg, round up, lift your head and bring your right knee over your right shoulder. If you can, bring your foot behind your head. If your foot doesn't go behind your head, place a block under your head. Hold and breathe. Switch sides and do the same thing on the other side.

This pose lengthens your low-back and helps your sacrum go back into alignment.

Standing Sacroiliac Joint Practice

You'll need your softball-sized ball and wall space.

Ball in your SI Joint at the Wall –

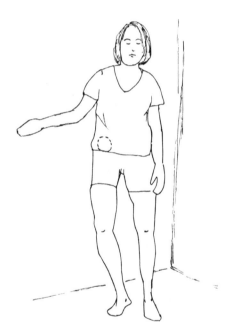

Come to a wall and place a ball right on the SI joint on the side that hurts. It will feel like you are on a swollen, often painful bump. Keep the ball here while you breathe slowly in and out for about thirty seconds. Move down on that same side to midway between the top of the sacrum and the tail, staying on the outer edge of the sacrum. Hold again for thirty seconds, then move down to just above your deep gluteal cleft (butt crack), the bottom of the sacrum, and hold again for thirty seconds.

Standing Lunge –

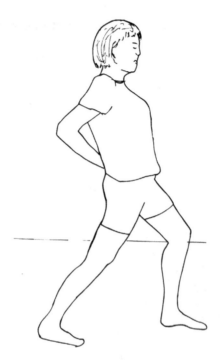

Stand with your feet inner hip-width apart, your feet parallel, and your knees softly bent. Drop your tail down, snap your ribs in and down, roll your inner arms out and squeeze your shoulder blades together. Step your foot back about two to three feet on the side your SI joint is out and bend your front knee until it is over your ankle.

Make a fist with the hand on the side the SI joint is out (the leg and foot that is behind you). As you exhale, press your fist into your SI joint. Inhale, release, then exhale and press. Do about five times, then hold and breathe.

You may have to do these practices several times a day to put the SI joint in and to get it to stay in!

Part IV: The Cure For Low-Back Pain – Maintenance

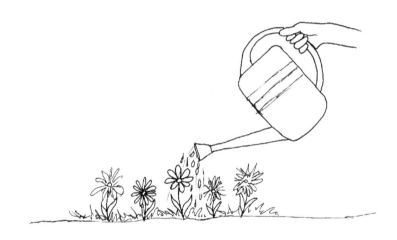

"I have so much to accomplish today that I must meditate for two hours instead of one." Mahatma Gandhi

Chapter 16 - How to Get Out of Low-Back Pain - Your Daily Practice

❀ DAILY PRACTICE ❀						
Sun	Mon	Tues	Wed	Thurs	Fri	Sat
		1	2	3	4	5
6	7	8	9	10	11	12
13	14	15	16	17	18	19
20	21	22	23	24	25	26
27	28	29	30	31		

"Practice is the hardest part of learning, and training is the essence of transformation."
Ann Voskamp

The key to your success is to maintain a daily practice every day. I recommend you do your daily practice as soon as you wake up in the morning.

I wake up, go to the bathroom, brush my teeth, put on my yoga pants and top, and get on my mat.

You have to maintain a daily practice because you are asking muscles that have a habit of hanging on, sometimes for decades, to let go. You developed your holding patterns over the years, and it takes consistent daily practice to remind your body that you really don't want your muscles to hang on in those ways anymore.

Remember that you are not only working on your physical body as you do your daily practice, you are telling your mind that you want to let go as well. The daily combination of working on your body and mind allows your whole being to get the message of how to hold your new Pain-Free Low-Back Posture.

Another reason the daily practice is best done in the morning is to ensure that you live your day in balance and alignment, using your new Pain-Free Low-Back Posture. If you start your day out of balance and alignment, you are far more likely to get in pain. So start your days all lined up!

Find a place in your home where you can have all of your balls, your mat, and other tools set up or easily accessible. I have a whole room devoted to my daily practice, and I leave out my mat and tools so that I can do my practice not only in the morning but whenever I need to.

Now, let's get you out of low-back pain!

Reminders:

- This is the Pain-Free Low-Back Daily Practice that has worked for the majority of my clients but if a certain ball work pose or movement doesn't work for you, just skip it and go on to the next movement. Everyone is unique in their low-back challenge.
- Never go into knee pain.
- While practicing, always breathe in through your nose and out through your mouth saying, *"Haaaa."*
- If your chin lifts while lying down, use a block or pillow under the back of your head.
- You can add into this Pain-Free Low-Back Daily Practice any of the ball work or movements from the previous practices that helped to release your low-back.

Pain-Free Low-Back Daily Practice

You'll need a yoga mat, Noodle Ball, softball-sized ball, golf ball, strap, block, and some wall space.

Ball Work - Low-Back Daily Practice

Ball in Your Iliopsoas and Quads –

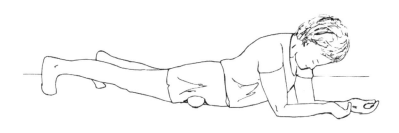

Lie on your belly. (This may hurt your low back initially. Keep doing it if the pain isn't too severe). Place a softball-sized ball to the inside of your right hip bone. Roll toward your pubic bone and back toward your hip bone. Your iliopsoas will be the place that feels a bit painful. Earlier I described the iliopsoas pain as feeling like a screechy violin. When you feel that, you know that you are in the right place.

Roll slowly down and into your inguinal crease (at the top of your leg, about halfway to your inner groin). The right iliopsoas represents fear of the outer world, others, and situations outside of yourself. Breathe out the fear and breathe in gratitude.

Keep rolling the ball down to your quads, across to the outer leg, back to the inner leg, and down to above your knee. The quads hold your fear response: flight, fight or freeze. Breathe out your held fear responses and breathe in freedom.

When ready, it's time to do the left side the same way that you did your right side, adding breathing out the fear of yourself and breathing in gratitude for your authentic self.

Ball in Your Inner Leg –

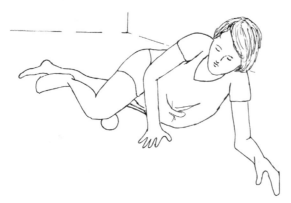

Place a softball-sized ball in your inner leg (groin area) in the graci-lis muscle. Move your leg up toward your chest and down toward your bottom as you roll down your inner leg to your knee. If you need to, place the ball up on a block. Breathe out anger. Switch sides and do the same thing on the other side.

This releases held anger that is stored in your inner legs. Dad teaches you how to deal with anger in the outer world (right side), and Mom teaches you how to handle anger within yourself (left side).

Softball-sized Ball in Your Butt Cheeks –

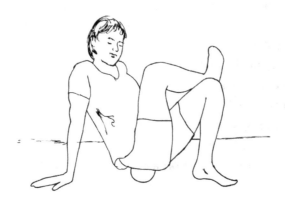

Lie down or sit up with the ball in your right butt cheek, with your right ankle on your left knee. Roll around finding knots of tension. Stay on the knots and move back and forth over them, breathing out control of others.

Switch sides after two minutes and place the ball in your left butt cheek, with your left ankle on your right knee. Roll around finding knots of tension. Stay on the knots and move back and forth over them, breathing out control of your inner world of feelings and intuition (which are your guidance system).

Noodle Ball Up Your Spine –

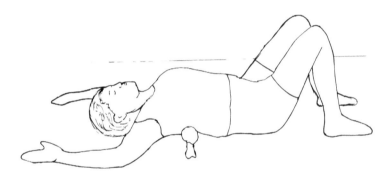

Place the Noodle Ball horizontally into your mid-butt cheeks. Rock side to side and slowly move up and into your low-back and mid-back, keeping your knees bent. Take your arms overhead as you move into your heart space. Continue moving up until the Noodle Ball falls off your shoulders.

A note from Pamela: *At first I hated the balls and Noodle Ball, but now they are my best friends. I take them everywhere I go, and I'm always looking for new balls to add to my collection.*

Stretches – Low-Back Daily Practice

Release your Quad and Iliopsoas Muscles –

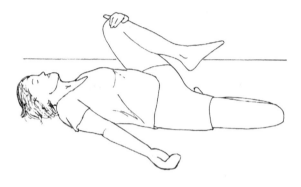

Lie on your back and hug both knees into your chest. Hold and breathe.

When ready, drop your right foot to the floor and walk it to the left, even with your left mid-butt cheek. Drop your right knee to the floor and pull your left knee to your chest.

Breathe out and brush off your fear responses to the outer world from your right thigh with your right hand as you exhale.

When ready, move your left leg around to go into different aspects of tension in your right quad muscles. Hold and breathe when in tight spaces.

To come out, hug both knees into your chest. Hold and breathe.

When ready, switch sides and do the same thing on the left side, adding breathing out and brushing off your fear responses from your inner world and left thigh with your left hand.

Butt Cheek Stretch —

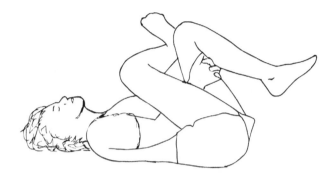

Lie on your back and place your right ankle on your left knee. Place your hands on the back of your left thigh and draw your left knee toward your chest. Find your edge (the end of your comfort zone; as far as you can go), then hold and breathe. Let go of control of your outer world and breathe in acceptance of whatever comes your way.

When ready, switch sides and place the left ankle on the right knee. On this side breathe out letting go of control of yourself and breathe in acceptance.

Lying Leg Opener –

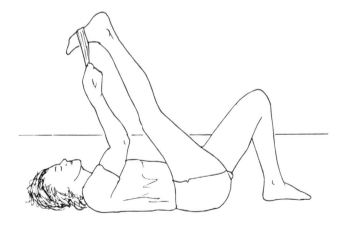

Lie on your back with your knees bent and your feet on the floor. Take your right knee to your chest and place a strap on the ball of your right foot. Inhale, bend your knee and exhale, extend through your heel opening the back of your leg. Do this several times until you are ready to hold.

As you hold, roll your inner leg in, press your heel to the sky, and take your toes down. With each exhalation, bring your thigh toward your belly until you reach the edge of the stretch in your hamstrings (the back of your leg). Hold and breathe.

When ready, place the strap in your right hand, keep your right leg straight and strong, and lower your right foot toward the floor to the right. Don't allow your pelvis on the left side to lift off the ground. Feel the stretch in your gracilis muscle (the inner leg) and breathe out anger as you hold the edge of this stretch.

When ready, exhale your straight, strong leg back to center, switch hands and bring your left hand on your strap. Exhale and bring your right foot to the left and your left knee to the right. Don't let your pelvis leave the floor on the right side. Feel the stretch in your IT band (the outer edge of your leg), hold the edge of this stretch, and breathe.

Come out, switch sides, and do the same thing on the other side.

This movement will open you to respect and appreciate your parents and to release what doesn't work for you from your upbringing.

Clock Pose –

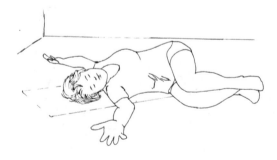

Lie on your back with your knees to your chest and keep them there as you roll over onto your right side. Take your arms out, even with your shoulders, and on an exhale bring your left arm overhead, keeping your fingertips on the floor. Inhale your arm back and exhale overhead three times, then hold and breathe in love!

Come out on an inhale and lie on your side for a couple of breaths, then flat on your back. Rest, switch sides, and do the same thing on the other side.

Hug Your Knees –

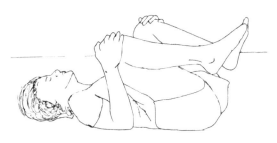

Lie on your back and bring your knees to your chest. Gently hug your knees and breathe deeply in and out of your belly. Feel your knees dropping into your body as you exhale and moving away from your body as you inhale. Rest here feeling the gentle rocking motion.

When ready, make circles slowly going in both directions. You can also rock gently from side to side. Breathe as you rock and/ or circle. **This pose can bring you a tremendous amount of relief from low-back pain.**

Strengtheners – Low-Back Daily Practice

Belly Strengthener at the Wall –

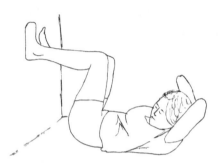

Place your feet on the wall at a right angle. Make sure your feet are lined up with your inner legs. Press into the outer edges of your heels as you lift your big toes. Feel the length of your low-back against the floor.

Put your right hand behind your left shoulder and your left hand behind your right shoulder, cradling your head. Breathe in and out of your belly. On an exhale lift up, taking your right elbow toward your left knee. Hold and breathe as long as you can. Come down on an exhale, and rest.

Switch sides by lifting up on an exhale and taking your left elbow toward your right knee. Hold and breathe, connecting to your power for as long as you can. Come down on an exhale, and rest. Do it as many times as you are comfortable.

Rest –

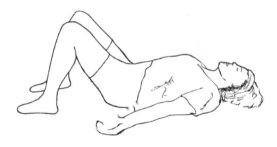

Lie on your back with your knees bent and your feet resting into the floor. Feel your lower back resting on the earth and breathe in and out of your pelvic bowl. Roll your inner arms out and rest them on the floor with your palms facing up. Soften your shoulders, move your head gently side to side and if your chin falls away from your chest, place a pillow behind your head. Go into stillness and feel your body breathing.

Low-Back Poses to Do Throughout the Day

Roll a Golf Ball on The Soles of Your Feet –

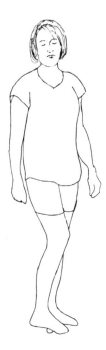

Stand on a golf ball and roll it around on the soles of your feet, finding knots of tension. Stay on the knots and breathe into your feet and out from your feet saying, *"Haaaa."* Focus on who brought you here into this life, your ancestors. Honor dad's ancestors as you roll on the bottom of your right foot. Honor your mom's ancestors as you roll on the bottom of your left foot.

Hip Opener on a Chair –

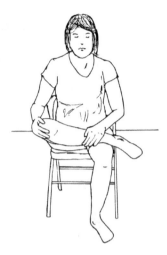

Sit on the edge of a chair and take your left ankle onto your right knee, flex your left foot and take your left hand above your left knee. Exhale, press your left knee down, inhale up, and keep going for about ten times. Then round forward, bringing your chest toward your calf. Hold and breathe out control. Come out, switch sides, and do the same thing on the other side.

Squats –

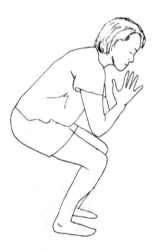

From standing, take your feet inner hip-width apart (or outer hip-width apart if you don't practice squats). Press into the outer edges of your heels, making sure your feet are facing straight ahead without ducking or pigeon-toeing.

Drop your tail and take your ribs in and down toward your pelvic bowl. Roll your inner arms out and squeeze your shoulder blades together.

Exhale out stress. Only bend your knees as far as you can — DO NOT go into knee pain!

Exhale down into a squat, inhale back up and continue. Build up to doing fifty squats a day.

Standing Hip and Butt Cheek Stretch —

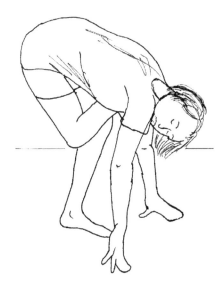

Stand next to a wall for balance. Stand into the left leg and take the right ankle on the left knee. Bend the standing leg as you fall forward, bringing your hands to the floor or a chair seat or wall.

Find your edge (the end of your comfort zone; as far as you can go) by bending the standing leg as much as you can and holding and breathing for two minutes. Breathe out control and breathe in acceptance.

Switch sides when ready

Standing Iliopsoas and Quad Release –

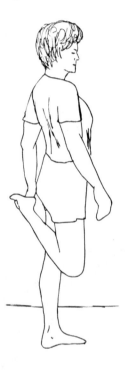

From standing, bring your weight onto your left foot, exhale and draw your right knee to your chest. Pause and feel the length of your lower back. Take your right hand down your shin as you drop your knee toward the floor.

Attempt to bring your knees even with one another while keeping a long lower back. Switch your grip to your left hand and bring your right heel toward your left buttocks.

Hold and breathe out fear. When ready, come back to standing, switch sides, and do the same thing on the other side.

Remember that the purpose of your daily practice is to familiarize yourself with your new Pain-Free Low-Back Posture! So, practice, practice, practice these essentials:

PAIN-FREE LOW-BACK POSTURE STANDING –

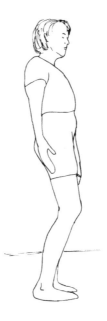

- Stand with your feet inner-hip width apart by lining up your feet, knees, and hips. (I place my hands to the inside of my hip bones, point my fingertips down and look down, lining up my feet with my hips, knees, and ankles).
- Make sure your feet are lined up and facing straight ahead.
- Press into the outer edges of your heels as you lift and spread your toes.
- Create a soft bend to your knees.
- Slightly roll your inner legs in.
- Pat out your butt cheeks to make sure that they are loose and free.
- Drop your tail and sacrum down as if beginning to sit in a chair.

- Lift your hip bones up.
- Draw your ribs in and down, which begins to work your abdominals.
- Roll your inner arms out.
- Squeeze your shoulder blades together and take them down toward your tail.
- Allow your head and neck to be loose and free.

As you try it, notice how the new Pain-Free Low-Back Posture feels. Remember, it will initially feel awkward because you are changing how you've stood since childhood.

PAIN-FREE LOW-BACK POSTURE WALKING –

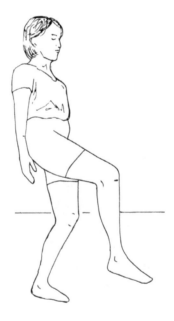

- Take the Pain-Free Low-Back Standing Posture detailed above.
- Sit back as if beginning to sit in a chair.
- Walk with your legs in front of you and your upper body sitting back loose and free.

PAIN-FREE LOW-BACK POSTURE SITTING –

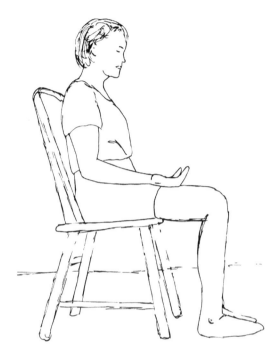

- Stand in front of a chair and take the Pain-Free Low-Back Standing Posture detailed above.
- Sit back as if sitting in the chair and keep going until you are actually sitting in the chair.
- As you sit, keep your tail down.
- Snap your ribs in and down.
- Roll your inner arms out, squeeze your shoulder blades together, and take them down toward your low-back.

Keep doing your daily practice and the Pain-Free Low-Back Posture will get easier and easier as your low-back feels better and better!

Oh, and best of all … you will soon get back to doing all of the things that you love to do!

A Pain-Free Low-Back Story –

I met Sandy when she couldn't walk to the bathroom and back because her sciatica pain was so severe. Sandy has horses and had been training them all summer when her sciatica began to act up.

I assessed Sandy's posture and could see tight piriformis (control) muscles, iliopsoas (fear) muscles, and lordosis (swayback). I gave Sandy her daily practice and Sandy says: *When I began my daily practice, I couldn't even walk to the bathroom; now, after just three weeks of doing my daily practice, I'm not only walking out to the barn and back up and down hills, but I'm also working with my horses again! It's a miracle.*

You, too, can experience a miracle!

Chapter 17 How to Stay Out of Low-Back Pain Facing Life Challenges

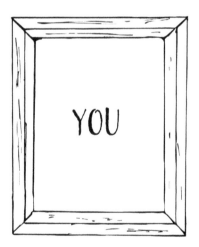

"Today, you have the opportunity to transcend from a disempowered mind-set of existence to an empowered reality of purpose-driven living. Today is a new day that has been handed to you for shaping. You have the tools, now get out there and create a masterpiece." — Steve Maraboli

As far as I can tell from taking this life journey for sixty years, we are put on this earth to face challenges and to overcome them. Because this is the nature of existence, I can easily predict that you will be challenged by life again and again.

And guess what?? Your old habitual low-back pain posture will return like an old friend, coming to help you out when you first encounter a life challenge.

Why? Well, think about it. You established your old painful low-back posture to protect yourself, and it worked for you – possibly for years. So your body's natural response to stressful life challenges is going to be to pull you back into that old painful posture. It thinks it is protecting you. It doesn't understand that this hurts you and causes your low-back pain.

So, as you face a stressful life situation, it is very important to **do your daily practice,** maybe even taking more time for it than you do on a normal day. Remember the saying from Gandhi that I shared earlier, *"I have so much to accomplish today that I must meditate for two hours instead of one."*

Gandhi knew that when life gave him a lot to handle, he had to double up on his daily practice. This is good advice for all of us!

Travel

So many of my clients make this mistake. But only once. They think: *I'm going on vacation, so I'll take a break from my daily practice. I don't want to carry my balls and movement tools with me.*

The reason they only make this mistake once is that when their low-back starts talking to them again while they're away, they sure wish that they'd packed their tools. They wish that they had a way to relieve this low-back pain because it is ruining their vacation.

Don't make this mistake. Take your balls and movement tools with you wherever you go. Bring a tennis ball with you in the car, on the train, or on the plane. I carry one in my purse at all times!

You can use the ball to get a good massage. My body is so used to getting a massage while I drive or ride in the car that if for some reason I don't have a ball with me, I've been known to use an apple or a water bottle to do the job. When I click on my seat belt, I reach for my ball and put it in my low-back, in my upper back, or under my butt cheek. Wherever my body says, *massage me here!*

Illness and Injury

We all get sick and injured no matter how careful we are, how well we eat, how many times we wash our hands, or how often we work out and do our daily practice. Sooner or later, something will get us. In times of illness or injury, do as much of the daily practice as you can.

One of my dear clients just had bladder surgery. As she recovered, she brought her balls into bed and did as much of the ball work and movements as she could. It not only helped her low-back stay out of pain; she believed it helped speed up her recovery.

Acceptance

This is my favorite quote on acceptance. *Acceptance is the answer to all my problems today. When I am disturbed, it is because I find some person, place, thing, or situation—some fact of my life—unacceptable to me, and I can find no serenity until I accept that person, place, thing, or situation as being exactly the way it is supposed to be at this moment. Nothing, absolutely nothing, happens in God's world by mistake. Unless I accept life completely on life's terms, I cannot be happy. I need to concentrate not so much on what needs to be changed in the world as on what needs to be changed in me and my attitudes.*

-The Big Book of Alcoholics Anonymous

This quote has helped me to release my low-back tension time and time again. When I remember that I didn't cause a situation, I can't change it, and I for sure can't control it, my butt cheeks soften and I take pressure off my low-back.

Acceptance for me is the definition of love. When I want someone to be different, I'm not loving them. If I want something to be different, I'm not coming from a place of love. If I want myself to be different, I'm not loving myself.

I know that this can be a difficult concept to grasp, because in some cases it seems that if you accept that person or thing, you are supporting it. But when we push against anything without accepting it, we are coming from a place of fear, anger, and control. And we will get fear, anger, and control coming right back toward us.

Now, if we come from a place of acceptance, we can find a way to work with the situation and guide it in the direction of love. We have the chance to find a solution that results in the best possible outcome for all.

A Pain-Free Low-Back Story –

Nora came to me with chronic low-back pain, sciatica, and a sacroiliac (SI) joint that was out of place. As we worked together, she shared her story, one of a lifetime of sexual abuse. Nora had just turned eighty, and a family member was still attempting to sexually abuse her.

As a result of all these decades of abuse, Nora's iliopsoas, piriformis, and gracilis muscles were all pulling her left hip bone into her hip socket, causing tremendous pain in her left hip, knee, and the left side of her low-back.

She began to take on this posture of protection when she was just eight years old. That is when she was first sexually abused by her stepdad. All these decades later, Nora was still posturing in this way – and it was hurting her every single day.

Nora began to work with me to release these tight muscles, and at the same time to accept what had happened to her (and what was still happening to her). She found the strength to set firm boundaries with her sexually abusive family member. Slowly, she also began to look at her abusers as teachers who had created a very strong woman, one who had helped to create programs in the prison system for sexual offenders.

Nora says: *My work with Michelle and my daily practice helped me to accept my fate, set healthy boundaries, and unravel my left leg from the tension of its protective hold. As I unwound, I began to relax more and more. As a result, angels seemed to come into my life to help and support me. I'm a work in progress at eighty years old. I'm so happy I lived long enough to do the work of letting go. My back, hip, and knee are happy too!*

I know that this work may not be a quick fix and at times can be challenging. But you can do it. You have the power to release your low-back pain, no matter what your age or circumstances, just like Nora did. You just needed to know what do to.

Now, you know.

Once you begin, I hope that you will maintain your daily practice, because as I said in my introduction ...

If you are alive, you can heal.

Thank you for reading my book. It is my mission to help as many people as possible find relief from low-back pain. I want to help you feel better because I know how it feels:

- to live with low-back pain.
- to try everything you can think of to release it.
- to give up hope of finding a way to resolve it.

Don't give up!!

If I can work my way out of low-back pain without pills, surgery, injections, or being popped or needled, you can work your way out as well.

If you follow the daily practice that I've outlined in this book for two months and your low-back pain does not reduce significantly, contact me at michelle@healthylowbackformula.com.

I've helped thousands of people release their low-back pain, and I'm here to help you too.

Here's to a healthy, happy low-back,
Michelle Andrie

References:

https://medium.com/the-ascent/3-steps-to-emotional-recovery-how-to-be-open-to-healing-2f8023fb5700

https://www.startstanding.org/back-pain-statistics-and-facts/#

https://www.buzzworthy.com/memories-dna-grandparents/

https://www.goodtherapy.org/blog/follow-your-heart-emotions-as-your-guidance-system-0818185

https://fs.blog/four-states-of-mind/

https://www.frontiersin.org/articles/10.3389/fpsyg.2020.01997/full

Tom Myers, the author of <u>Anatomy Trains</u>.

<u>Understanding your Fascia</u> by Julia Lucus

<u>The Structure That Carries Consciousness</u> featured in the May/June 2016 edition of Energy Magazine, author: Marisa Chadbourne, LMT, JFB Myofascial Therapist

Cardiologist Bruno Bordoni who wrote the article <u>The Awareness of the Fascial System</u>

https://kidshealth.org/

https://edenenergymedicine.com/

https://www.healthline.com/health/what-is-an-aura

https://www.sciencedirect.com/topics/medicine-and-dentistry/body-meridian

https://www.forbes.com/health/body/what-is-reiki/

https://www.freeletics.com/en/blog/posts/human-energy-systems-beginners-guide/

https://anodeajudith.com/

https://barbarabrennan.com/

CPSIA information can be obtained
at www.ICGtesting.com
Printed in the USA
LVHW021931120423
744168LV00001B/158

9 781958 848531